CAREERS

How to get a specialty training post: the insider's guide

SUCCESS IN MEDICINE SERIES

How to get a specialty training post: *the insider's guide*

WRITTEN BY

Danny C.G. Lim, MBBS, BSc, MRCP

Cardiology Specialty Trainee,
Northern Deanery,
Queen Elizabeth Hospital,
Gateshead, UK

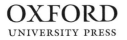

OXFORD
UNIVERSITY PRESS

OXFORD

UNIVERSITY PRESS

Great Clarendon Street, Oxford OX2 6DP

Oxford University Press is a department of the University of Oxford.
It furthers the University's objective of excellence in research, scholarship,
and education by publishing worldwide in

Oxford New York

Auckland Cape Town Dar es Salaam Hong Kong Karachi
Kuala Lumpur Madrid Melbourne Mexico City Nairobi
New Delhi Shanghai Taipei Toronto

With offices in

Argentina Austria Brazil Chile Czech Republic France Greece
Guatemala Hungary Italy Japan Poland Portugal Singapore
South Korea Switzerland Thailand Turkey Ukraine Vietnam

Oxford is a registered trade mark of Oxford University Press
in the UK and in certain other countries

Published in the United States
by Oxford University Press Inc., New York

© Oxford University Press, 2011

British Library Cataloguing in Publication Data
Data available

Library of Congress Cataloging in Publication Data
Data available

Typeset in Charter by Glyph International, Bangalore, India
Printed in Great Britain
on acid-free paper by
CPI Antony Rowe, Chippenham, Wiltshire

ISBN 978–0–19–959080–3

10 9 8 7 6 5 4 3 2 1

To my dad for teaching me the importance of working hard and smart.

To my mum for encouraging me to always strive further.

To my wife for her unwavering love and support.

Acknowledgements

Thanks to Fiona Goodgame for taking the time to listen to a new, untested author. I must also thank Katy Loftus and Christopher Reid for their indispensable advice in writing this book. Philippa Hendry and her team have brought this book to life.

My gratitude to contributors Christopher Lamb, Anthony Jesurasa, Benjamin Morton, and Simon Wan for their suggestions.

Contents

Specialty advisors

Ahmed Al-Maskari
OPHTHALMOLOGY

Rachael Elizabeth Baines
PLASTIC SURGERY

Vish Battacharya
INTERVIEW

Claire Bell
PAEDIATRICS

Gemma Conn
GENERAL SURGERY

Helen Cooper
ACUTE MEDICINE

Clare Ginnis
EMERGENCY MEDICINE

Benedict Hayhoe
GENERAL PRACTICE

Catherine Houlihan
INFECTIOUS DISEASE

Aisha Janjua
OBSTETRICS & GYNAECOLOGY

Amrita Jesurasa
PUBLIC HEALTH

Anthony Jesurasa
NEUROSURGERY

Ayesha Khan
GENERAL SURGERY

Jeremy Killen
INTERVIEW

Mary Ann Kwok
GENERAL PRACTICE

Christopher Lamb
GASTROENTEROLOGY

Adrian Lim
CMT

Alice Lomax
PSYCHIATRY

Frances Marr
RENAL MEDICINE

Cara Marshall
ACCS: ANAESTHETICS

Benjamin Mortin
ANAESTHETICS

Akash Patel
TRAUMA & ORTHOPAEDICS

Preethi Rao
DIABETES AND ENDOCRINOLOGY

Bervin Teo
ACCS

Vik Veer
ENT

Simon Wan
RADIOLOGY

CHAPTER I

The 'secret' to getting into specialty training

Don't just work hard, work smart

Introduction

Who gets the job?

This may surprise you, but the doctor most likely to get a training job is not necessarily the best or most knowledgeable clinician. So, what are the deaneries looking for?

The doctor most likely to succeed fulfils the selection criteria and can demonstrate it! It is the combination of having a great product and a great sales pitch that is most likely to succeed.

The book I wish I had had

In this book, I will reveal precisely how deaneries evaluate applicants at short-listing and interview. In the past, I have found it difficult to get hold of this information.

The advice in this book is based on multiple sources. From deanery and royal college websites I have sourced over a hundred short-listing protocols and dozens of interview scoring systems. In addition, over 20 specialty trainees, all from different specialties, have contributed to it. Consultants with years of interview experience have also contributed to the chapters on interview.

Use this book as your 'traveller's guide' on your journey to specialty training. I hope it will give you the guidance that I wish I had had when I was applying for training jobs.

Working smart

Don't be like a hamster running round a spinning wheel. Sure, the hamster is working hard, but it's getting nowhere! Hard work is essential, but it needs to be strategic. For example, if you were a Foundation Year (FY) doctor aspiring to be a surgeon, studying a giant textbook of surgery from cover to cover would be pointless. From a career perspective, your free time would be better spent on areas the selection process looks at—this could be an audit, a case report, or a research project.

The amount of effort you dedicate to working on your CV (*curriculum vitae*) will have a tremendous impact on your chances of securing a training post. In **CHAPTER 2** I will reveal tips and what you need to work on to get ahead.

The selection process

There are four hurdles you need to overcome: application submission, long-listing, short-listing, and interviews (or selection centre).

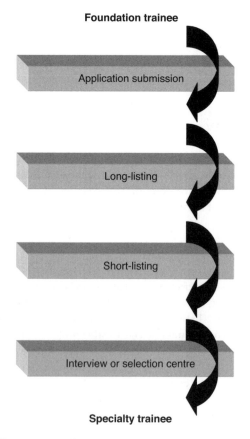

Foundation trainee

Application submission

Long-listing

Short-listing

Interview or selection centre

Specialty trainee

Figure 1.1 A diagrammatic representation of the selection process.

Application submission

For most specialties, the main application period is short and takes place once a year. Deaneries can advertise a job for only 3 days and can give you as little as 5 days to submit your application. You need to know when and where to apply or wait for another year. **CHAPTER 3** gives more information about being ready to apply.

Long-listing

After submitting your application form, selectors will first check that you fulfil all the essential criteria. This should be straightforward provided you've done your homework. The next step is short-listing.

Short-listing

The bigger specialties receive several thousand job applications annually. It is not feasible (or possible!) to interview every single applicant. Short-listing serves to separate the wheat from the chaff.

Most specialties short-list with application forms. Each response on the application form is marked according to a pre-defined marking scheme. The marking scheme is based on the person specifications. The total score for each candidate's application form makes up the short-listing score. Only the highest scoring candidates get invited to interview.

An alternative is to short-list using a selection exam. General Practice and Public Health are the only major specialties that use exams at the time of writing. However, other specialties are planning to use selection exams in the not too distant future, particularly for CT1–2 level. In 2010, ACCS (Acute Care Common Stem), Anaesthetics, Histopathology, Medicine, Paediatrics, and Psychiatry piloted the use of selection exams. In anticipation of this, there is a section on selection exams—**CHAPTER 4** covers application forms and selection exams.

Interview or selection centre

If you've made it to this stage, then you're one step away from your goal. Statistically, you have a one in four chance of getting the post.

For most specialties, interview is still part of selection. However, many specialties now incorporate additional forms of assessment. Role-playing scenarios, group discussions, practical skills assessment, telephone exercises, and presentation stations are just a few of the many tasks of you could encounter at a selection centre.

Your performance at interview or in any of these tasks is evaluated with a highly structured marking scheme. Emphasis is placed on objectivity, and assessors have to undergo training beforehand. The total score you achieve at interview is then combined (in variable ways) with your short-listing score. It is this final score that determines if you will be offered a training post.

CHAPTERS 5 AND 6 are dedicated to interviews and selection centres. **CHAPTER 7** is crammed with specific advice for each major specialty.

CHAPTER 2

Career development: the secret of success

Luck favours the prepared   **Louis Pasteur**

This is arguably the most important chapter of the book. An athlete wins an Olympic gold medal because of outstanding performance on race day. But this performance was possible only because of years of sweat and tears beforehand. Likewise, your application form and interview performance determine your chances of securing a training post. This is ultimately determined by the effort you have invested in developing your career over the preceding years. Some claim that you need to be lucky to get a training post. To a large extent, you make your own luck.

Key points about career development

- **Start early.** This is important. Research projects, audits, exams, presentations, and publications require months to years to complete. Applications for many training posts open half a year in advance.
- **Start, even if you are uncertain about your specialty.** With the exception of General Practitioner (GP), there is a tremendous amount of overlap in the selection criteria. An audit, prize, or publication usually scores you points even if it is in a different specialty. So, there is no excuse to stop you writing up that case report!

- **Go the extra mile.** To build an outstanding portfolio you need to do more than the minimum. For example, instead of just doing your bit for an audit, why not offer to lead it, propose changes, present it, and, if appropriate, submit the abstract to conferences and journals. Likewise, publications are not compulsory for Foundation year (FY) doctors, but if you manage to get published in a peer-reviewed journal then you will have a head-start.
- **Be all-rounded, work on weak areas.** Many selection processes will eliminate applicants who perform poorly in particular areas. For example, if you have never participated in an audit before make this your next priority. Use the development tool on **(PAGE 9)** in this chapter to identify weak areas.

Which specialty?

Only you can answer this question. I recommend doing your research and taking your time. There are several factors you have to consider:

Your interest. You have to be interested in the specialty. This is a decision that will affect you for the rest of your working life; you have to enjoy it. If you have a strong interest in a specialty, your chances of a successful career increase. You would be more inclined to get involved in projects such as research, audits, and publications. At interview, experienced interviewers will detect your enthusiasm (or lack of it) for the specialty.

Lifestyle. Regular versus unsociable hours. Are there opportunities for part-time work? If you strongly dislike working unsociable hours, then you would be unhappy in Emergency or Critical Care Medicine. Likewise, if spending time with your family is a priority, consider specialties where part-time work is readily available such as General Practice.

Competitiveness. If you are applying to a very competitive specialty, you have to be prepared to dedicate considerable time on career development and perhaps years in research. Realistically, you are going to have to be geographically flexible. This could have major implications, particularly if you have a family or mortgage. Be sure you are willing to make such sacrifices.

Earnings. Money is important, even for doctors. For some specialties private work will be non-existent.

If you are undecided, here are a few suggestions:

- MedicalCareers.nhs.uk is a great place to start. It has lots of practical advice, personality tests, and information on a variety of specialties to consider (www.medicalcareers.nhs.uk)
- The BMJ group regularly organizes careers fairs which give you the opportunity to talk to trainees and consider different career pathways (www.careersfair.bmj.com).

- For more information on different specialties, *So you want to be a brain surgeon*, edited by Simon Eccles and Stephan Sanders (3rd edn, Oxford University Press, 2009) is an excellent source.

Your development score

Table 2.1 contains a self-assessment tool that you can use to monitor your career development. The career development tool incorporates objective criteria that are commonly gauged at short-listing or interview. It assumes that you have fulfilled all the essential criteria. You can use it in the following ways:

1. An estimate of your 'desirability' in the eyes of selectors. The higher the score, the more employable you are.

Table 2.1 A self-assessment tool for monitoring career development

Selection criteria	Scoring key	Score	Key
Postgraduate degrees	**Maximum 8**		
PhD	8		≥6 Above
MD	6		average
MPhil	6		3–5 OK, but
BSc 1st class	6		room for
MSc	4		improve-
BSc 2:1	3		ment
BSc Other	2		≤2 Area of
			weakness
Royal College exam	**Maximum 10**		
Full membership	8		<2 Area of
1st part	2		weakness
2nd part	2		
Prizes	**Maximum 6**		
International or national prize	6		≥4 Above
Prize awarded as part of final MB	5		average
Prize awarded as part of undergraduate course	4		3 OK, but room for
Scholarships or bursaries for medical school	2		improve- ment
Other undergraduate or postgraduate prizes	2		≤2 Area of weakness

➲

Audit and clinical governance	**Maximum 10**	
Presented audit at international or national meeting	4	≥7 Above average
Presented audit at regional meeting	3	5–6 OK, but room for improve-ment
Presented audit at local meeting	2	
Re-audit or closed cycle	2	
Changes or recommendations made	2	
Completed an audit	2	≤4 Area of weakness
Completed critical incident form	2	
Presentation	**Maximum 6**	
International meeting	6	≥5 Above average
National meeting	5	
Regional meeting	4	3–4 OK, but room for improve-ment
Poster presentation (any meeting)	4	
Local meeting	2	≤2 Area of weakness
Publications	**Maximum 8**	
1st author for major peer-reviewed publication	5	≥6 Above average
1st author for peer-reviewed publication	4	3–5 OK, but room for improve-ment
Co-author for peer-reviewed publication	3	
Published abstract	2	≤2 Area of weakness
Published article (not peer-reviewed)	2	
Teaching	**Maximum 8**	
Designed and led regional programme plus formal training	6	≥6 Above average
Designed and led regional programme	4	3–5 OK, but room for improve-ment
Designed local programme plus formal training	4	
Designed local programme	2	
Regular participation in local programme (i.e. weekly)	2	≤2 Area of weakness
Occasional participation in teaching	1	
Training courses	**Maximum 5**	
Attendance at specialty-relevant course (compulsory courses do not count)	2	≤2 Area of weakness

➲

Commitment to specialty	Maximum 16	
Relevant research project	4	≥11 Above average
Attendance at professional society conference	4	7–10 OK, but room for improve-ment
Previous or current post in specialty	3	
Presentation relating to specialty at major conference	3	
Publication relating to specialty	3	
Attendance at relevant conference or seminar	2	≤6 Area of weakness
Spoken at depth with multiple trainees about specialty	2	
Regular reading of specialty journal	2	
Audit relating to specialty	2	
Effort to gain additional shadowing experience	2	
Taster week (if no specialty experience)	1	
Presentation relating to specialty at local conference	1	
Paper portfolio (to bring to interview)	**Maximum 10**	
Divided into different sections with index page	2	≥7 Above average
Chronologically arranged and organized	2	5–6 OK, but room for improve-ment
Complete with audits, presentations, publications etc.	2	
Complete logbook of practical skills (if relevant)	2	≤4 Area of weakness
Evidence of regular reflective practice (monthly or more)	2	
Personal development plan	2	
ST3+ applicants only	**Maximum 12**	
PhD, MD or MPhil related to specialty	4	≥9 Above average
Multiple skills relevant to specialty (DOPS or certificate)	4	5–8 OK, but room for improve-ment
LAT or LAS post	4	
Trust grade or clinical fellow	2	
Acquired a skill relevant to specialty (DOPS or certificate)	2	≤4 Area of weakness
	Total	

DOPS, Direct Observation of Procedural Skills; LAT, locum appointment for training; LAS, locum appointment for service.

2. Monitor your career development and chart your progress on your path to specialty training. For example, if your total score is 16, you can set yourself a target of 20 in 6 months' time.
3. Identifying weak areas. If your score is particularly low in specific areas, you can work on this.

How to use the development tool

- Award yourself a score for every criterion you fulfil.
- You can add up scores for each selection criterion.
- There is a maximum score for each selection criterion.
- The grand total is your development score.

Prizes

Your best chance of winning a prize is as a medical student, simply because of the sheer number of prizes to be won. Prizes come in the form of bursaries and for essay competitions and presentations. Students can even win bursaries to attend open days and conferences! Junior doctors can still win prizes, mainly in the form of research or presentation prizes.

The first hurdle before winning a prize is to identify one. Here are a few tips on where to look:

- rdfunding.org.uk is a good site to search for prizes according to specialty. Make sure you limit your search to prizes only.
- The Royal Society of Medicine (RSM) website (www.rsm.ac.uk) lists dozens of awards in a variety of specialties including Surgery, Pathology, Psychiatry, and Paediatrics. Definitely worth a visit.
- The relevant royal college and specialty society websites usually have information on prizes and fellowships.
- **CHAPTER 7** will have more suggestions for each specialty. In addition to your specialty, look at related specialties too. For example, a budding respiratory physician can also look under General Medicine, Geriatrics, and Intensive Care Medicine.

Medical students have tonnes of opportunities to win bursaries, elective grants, and essay prizes!

Bursaries

Bursaries count as prizes. Most royal colleges and societies award bursaries to students organizing an elective or project related to the relevant specialty. The awards are made annually and they are always worth trying for—plus the spare cash will come in handy. There are also bursaries for attending conferences and these will look good on any CV. Read **CHAPTER 7** for details of bursaries according to specialty.

Essay prizes

Many royal colleges and specialty societies host annual essay competitions for medical students and junior doctors. I recommend visiting the websites of these societies to look for such awards. In addition, the RSM hosts numerous essay competitions in a variety of specialties each year. Writing a several thousand word essay won't take long and could be a big boost to your CV.

Presentation prizes

I would encourage all junior doctors to submit abstracts to conferences. You might get selected to give an oral or poster presentation. There is usually a prize for outstanding presentations and sometimes there is a prize allocated to trainees. Read the next section on Presentations for more information.

Research prizes

You can submit your research findings at numerous competitions hosted by royal colleges and professional societies. These societies also award annual fellowships and grants for research which can be counted as prizes. The RSM also hosts research competitions in a variety of specialties.

Presentations

Most junior doctors will have given a local presentation at work. Few take it up a level and therefore miss out on a big CV boost.

Local presentations

Most hospitals have a programme of grand rounds or educational half-days. There are also departmental meetings and journal clubs. These are all opportunities to build up your CV. Ask your consultant for an opportunity to present the next time it's your team's turn. You could contact the person in charge of organizing such meetings for potential opportunities. Some hospitals also host a presentation competition for trainee doctors. Look out for these.

If you already have a few local presentations under your belt, switch your focus to regional, national, or international presentations. More local presentations aren't going to increase your short-listing score—the law of diminishing returns.

Regional presentations

Regional presentations carry more weight than local ones. Approach the relevant consultant for opportunities to present at the next regional meeting. Alternatively, contact the educational director for the specialty for suggestions.

National and international conferences

Most specialist societies host annual (or biannual) conferences. For the majority of conferences there is a call for abstracts of poster or oral presentations to be made at the meeting. In **CHAPTER 7** I list the opportunities for presentations for each specialty. Don't forget to consider related organizations too. For example, if you are a wannabe plastic surgeon, you can present to plastic surgery societies, the Royal College of Surgeons, and the RSM.

Presenting at such meetings ticks many career boxes and is strongly recommended. A national or international presentation carries much more weight at short-listing and can be an impressive talking point at interview. It proves your commitment to the specialty. Abstracts are usually published in the relevant society's peer-reviewed journal. Plus, if your presentation goes down well, you could win a prize.

Don't be intimidated, you may be pleasantly surprised at the number of presentations being accepted annually. Poster presentations are much more likely to be successful because much larger numbers can be accepted, so they are worth a shot. Oral presentations are harder to get accepted but if you do succeed it will be particularly impressive. If you have a good topic to present, it is worth an attempt.

Read the rules on what material is accepted, i.e. audits, research, case reports. Check who is allowed to present. Some conferences allow anybody attending to submit, but others require a member to co-present.

Publications

Being published is advantageous at many levels. It will give you a boost at short-listing and your publications can be a handy talking point at interview. A string of decent publications will grab the attention of any interview panel. Publications also demonstrate your commitment to the specialty and bolster your credibility as an applicant.

Here are a few myths I want to dispel:

1. **It is difficult for junior doctors and medical students to get published.**
   Nonsense! There are journals that encourage submissions from medical students and junior doctors. It requires some thought and work, but it's definitely doable.

2. **Research is the best way to get published.** From the point of view of a job application this is not necessarily true; it depends on your time-scale. If you are applying for jobs in a year or less it is unlikely that a research project would result in publications by then. In this section are a few alternative routes to getting published.

3. **Only peer-reviewed publications count.** Publications in newspapers, newsletters, or magazines would show your interest in the specialty and still impress interviewers. It would also be more impressive than a blank section on your application form. You can list such articles in the publications section unless specified otherwise.

4. **Publications must be in your specialty.** As far as most short-list marking schemes are concerned, there is no difference in the score allocated. Considering other areas opens up your options.

A book I have found extremely useful to getting published is *The complete guide to medical writing* edited by Mark Stuart (Pharmaceutical Press, 2007).

Newsletters, local newspapers, or magazines

Widen your scope and write an article in a local newspaper or magazine. Medical newsletters such as JuniorDr.com and HospitalDr.co.uk are alternatives. Such articles take less time to be accepted for publication.

Browse through the abovementioned publications. If you have an idea, e-mail the editor and suggest an article. Try to combine your interests. For example, I was a keen recreational runner and also interested in Cardiology. I e-mailed editors of running magazines and proposed an article on running and sudden cardiac death. One editor liked my idea and within a few months I had an article in a national magazine.

'Letters to the editor' or responses

Have you ever had a thought or point to raise when reading an article in a journal? Why not submit your response to the editor. Online journals allow you to submit your response on their website. Your response could be selected for inclusion in the online or print edition. Your name could appear within a few weeks (even faster if online). An alternative is to submit a Letter to the Editor on a published article. If your letter is interesting, it may get published in the next issue.

Case reports

Case reports are quick to write up, but getting one published in a major journal is difficult because of the competition. Your case report is more likely to get published if you submit it to a journal dedicated to case reports.

1. **BMJ Case Reports**: peer-reviewed online journal (Medline indexing pending). It is a sister-publication to the *BMJ* and aims to 'publish a high

volume of cases in all disciplines'. To submit a case report, you have to pay an annual fee of £95 (as of October 2010). In my opinion, that is money well spent.

2. **JRSM Short Reports**: peer-reviewed online journal launched by the RSM in 2010. It is PubMed Central indexed. There is a publication fee of £350 per accepted article (as of October 2010).

3. **Journal of Medical Case Reports**: an online, peer-reviewed, PubMed Central indexed journal. It publishes dozens of case reports each month from all specialties. There is an article processing fee of £550 (as of May 2010).

Review papers

Choose a focused specialty area that interests you and write a review article. You would need to define the scope of the article and perform a thorough literature search. It helps if you can get a consultant to be your co-author and review the article before submission. *British Journal of Hospital Medicine*, *British Journal of Medical Practitioners*, and *Geriatric Medicine* are journals that specialize in reviews.

Forget-me-not journals

If you were rejected by the *New England Journal of Medicine* why not submit to a less famous journal? Sure, it may have a lower impact factor, but you will still earn valuable short-listing points. Setting your sights a little lower will improve your odds of acceptance, open up more journals to submit to, and there could be less competition.

Keep an eye out for such journals in your hospital library. You can also browse PubMed's journal list categorized by specialty (wwwcf.nlm.nih.gov/serials/journals/index.cfm). Below are a few suggestions to get you started:

1. The *Foundation Years Journal*: a peer-reviewed journal that accepts case-based articles, reviews, research, and audit. Articles written by junior doctors of all grades will be considered.

2. BioMed Central publishes over 200 online journals, covering almost every specialty. Because of their online format, a greater number of articles may be published. Case reports, original research, reviews, and commentaries are accepted. The only catch is that there is an article processing fee, typically about £1000.

3. Regional journals. *The West London Medical Journal* and *The Darlington & County Durham Medical Journal* are just two examples. Browse your hospital library for more ideas.

Journals in non-clinical areas

This is an alternative (and much forgotten) way of getting published in a peer-reviewed journal. Consider writing an article in areas such as medical history, biography, education, ethics, or law. For example, a budding surgeon could write an article on the historical management of appendicitis. Below are a few suggestions:

- Medical history: *Journal of Medical Biography, Journal of the History of Medicine and Allied Sciences, Bulletin of the History of Medicine.*
- Education: *Postgraduate Medical Journal, Medical Teacher, Journal of Medical Education.*
- Ethics and law: *Medico-Legal Journal, Clinical Ethics.*

Professional examinations

I strongly recommend sitting professional exams early on, especially if you know what your specialty interest is. Passing professional exams is solid proof of your commitment to the specialty. It also helps your short-listing score and the interview panel are more likely to take you seriously.

It is expected that clinical problem-solving tests will be used to select candidates. Studying for professional exams will give you an advantage and get you into exam mode. Many Core Medical Training (CMT) applicants who sat the pilot selection exam remarked on the similarity it had to the MRCP exam.[1]

In the past, FY doctors were advised by deanery staff against sitting professional exams. For the benefits outlined above, I suggest disregarding this advice. Many FY doctors who followed this advice are now unhappy with it. Ask your seniors about the appropriate exam for you and ensure that you are eligible to enrol.

Exam preparation

The most time-efficient way to prepare is to practice lots of past questions. There are many websites and books that let you practice questions for a small (and worthwhile) fee. Your aim is to practice thousands of these questions repeatedly. Learn from your mistakes and read up areas of weakness in your textbook. Most successful candidates use practice questions and few recommend revising directly from reference books.

Know your full study leave entitlement and make full use of it. If you can, attend a reputable revision course. Going on such courses gives you time off to concentrate on your revision. Observing how much other delegates know will frighten you into studying! Apply for private study leave too; the few extra days off the wards will help.

Commitment to the specialty

Clinical experience

Ideally, you should have experience in the specialty; this is the best way to learn it. Apply for rotations that feature your specialty early on: you will learn about the pros and cons of the specialty and you are more likely to get ideas for research, audits, and publications. There will be opportunities to observe clinics and practical procedures. Trainees will give you advice on applying for jobs and building your CV. Talking to consultants and trainees will teach you how to 'talk the talk': a study by Peninsula Deanery showed that FY applicants to CT1 in Surgery fared better in interviews if they had already worked in the Foundation Year.[2]

Tasters

An alternative to a clinical post is to organize a 'tasters' week. Make the most of your week and keep a diary to record your experiences; this will come in handy when preparing for interview. Talk to trainees and consultants as much as you can. Ask them about the training and their likes and dislikes in the specialty. Ask their advice on conferences to attend and exams to sit.

In addition to tasters, negotiate with your educational supervisor regular sessions shadowing your specialty of interest, i.e. attending theatres and outpatients.

Research your specialty

Research the specialty well. There is a wealth of information online. Visit the relevant royal college's website and find out about the training structure and career pathway. The Modernising Medical Careers (MMC) website (www.mmc.nhs.uk) has information about competition ratios and person specifications. BMJCareers (careers.bmj.com) is a good website containing career guidance on different specialties. Finally, take every opportunity to talk to trainees and consultants.

Society membership and conferences

Every specialty will have societies which you should join and become involved with. There is usually an annual conference which I recommend you attend. Even better, submit an abstract to present at the conference.

Courses and seminars

In addition to conferences, most societies and royal colleges organize courses and seminars. You will get a certificate for attending and can talk about it at interview. Students and doctors in training often pay a discounted fee.

Publications, audit, research, and presentations

Participating in these would be further proof of your commitment. Read the relevant sections in this chapter for more advice.

Keep up to date

Build up your knowledge base and keep up with topical issues in the specialty by reading relevant journals in the library regularly. If you can afford it, a subscription is a worthwhile investment. Journals will also advertise prizes, conferences, and seminars.

Audit

Every junior doctor should have one good audit on their CV, and if you haven't you should make this a priority. Quality is more important than quantity. What defines a quality audit? Here are the criteria that selectors are looking for:

1. **Self-initiated, or coordinated by the applicant.** Approach your consultant and discuss your proposal for an audit. Choose a straightforward audit that can be completed quickly. Offer to take charge of the project, with them overseeing it.
2. **Self-designed audit.** Taking charge of the audit means you can design it and devise your own criteria. You can also design a data collection proforma.
3. **Findings were presented.** On completion of your audit, suggest that you present your findings at the next departmental meeting or grand round.
4. **Recommendations or guidelines were made.** It's worthwhile spending some time pondering on your findings. What recommendations can you make? Why not draft trust-wide guidelines based on your findings? Write up your proposals and suggest them to your consultant.
5. **The audit cycle was closed.** Junior doctors usually move hospitals, so this can be tricky. Try to keep in contact with your audit consultant. Offer to assist in any re-audit at a later date, perhaps in an advisory role. At the very least, find out about the results of any re-audit so that you can talk about this at interview. An alternative is to participate in a re-audit.
6. **A final flourish.** If your audit was particularly good, try presenting it at a conference, or consider submitting it for publication in the *Foundation Years Journal*. If you have already completed an audit ensure you have presented it at a meeting. If the findings were significant, you should consider presenting it at a regional grand round or regional meeting. Discuss this with the consultant in charge.

Research

What you will get out of research depends on what you make of it. A good research project will be a major boost on your journey to a specialty training post. The experience itself will provide you with insights into research. If you are awarded a grant, fellowship, or postgraduate degree this is a plus on your CV. Your results can be presented at conferences or be published. There are potential prizes for outstanding research and presentations.

Research project

Getting involved in a research project part-time can be done whilst working full-time, though dedication is a must. In my experience, whatever hospital you go to, if people know you are interested there are always projects available. Ask around and speak to consultants who have research interests. They often love to hear from enthusiastic trainees who want to get involved.

If this is your first research project, be realistic and avoid overly ambitious projects. Your first project should ideally be straightforward with a limited timescale. Database or literature-based projects can be relatively straightforward and performed in your spare time. Cell or animal-based research projects usually require daily laboratory visits (including weekends!). Research with animal and human studies may require Home Office or ethical approval, prolonging the entire project.

UK Comprehensive Clinical Research Network (CLRN)

Get involved in UK CLRN work. It's a way to make UK trial recruitment attractive and accessible to all clinicians and not just those in central teaching hospitals. Again juniors could get involved in data collection etc. (see www.crncc.nihr.ac.uk).

Fellowships, MDs, PhDs

The downside of MDs or PhDs is that they require years out of clinical practice with the accompanying loss of skill and earnings. However, if you can make the most of your research, the rewards you'll reap are well worth it.

Securing funding for any research is the first challenge. Royal colleges, professional societies, and charities all award research fellowships and grants. Search the relevant websites. An alternative is to search rdfunding.org.uk for potential sources of funds.

Teaching

This is a much neglected part of the CV for many doctors, which is a shame as it only requires a little effort to polish. Most doctors will have done some impromptu teaching, but to stand out, I suggest the following.

Provide evidence

When you next teach at a grand round or an educational session, distribute evaluation forms to your audience. Such forms can be downloaded from the JRCPTB (Joint Royal Colleges of Physicians Training Board) website (www.jrcptb.org.uk). Collect their feedback and add this to your portfolio. You have now been peer-evaluated as a teacher (a plus at shortlisting) and can use this in future application forms.

Be trained to teach

Get formal training in teaching skills and techniques. This will boost your shortlisting score and be an additional talking point at interview. There are many such courses, for example Teaching Skills For Doctors (RSM), On-The-Job Teaching (Royal College of Physicians, RCP), Teach the Teacher (Apply2Medicine, Oxford Medical).

Have a formal teaching role

Approach the educational director for undergraduates or foundation year doctors at your hospital. Offer your time to teach as part of the educational programme. Keep an eye out for e-mails asking for volunteers to teach and jump at such opportunities. If you have contributed to an educational website, this is another role worth mentioning.

If you have been forwarded as instructor at a resuscitation course you have a great opportunity to boost your teaching and leadership profile. I strongly recommend you complete the training to instructor level.

Be course director

Designing or coordinating a teaching programme will attract high marks in short-listing. Why not create your own course? This is not as crazy as it sounds, and is doable. Your achievement can also be used to demonstrate your leadership and management experience in other parts of the application form. From personal experience, creating and running a course can be a very rewarding experience.

Below is a suggested route for designing your own course. Chose a topic that you are confident in, e.g. history taking, examination skills, X-rays and ECG interpretation. Recruit a few like-minded colleagues and together design a course timetable for medical students. It could be a Saturday course or a once-a-week evening course depending on your commitments. Assign specific roles for each tutor involved. Negotiate a venue with the medical school or education centre in your hospital.

Advertise your course to medical students via posters in the medical school and hospital notice boards. Alternatively, ask if the medical school administrator could e-mail details of your course to the students. You could charge a fee to cover costs but do make sure it is affordable! Set a strict limit on the number of students on the course.

On the course day, make sure you have feedback forms to let you know how the students found it. Keep the feedback forms and your course timetable for your portfolio as proof of your teaching. Last, but not least, don't forget to enjoy the whole experience!

Portfolio

Expect your portfolio to be scrutinized and graded at interview. This takes place for the majority of specialties. The score from your portfolio station can account for up to a third of the interview score, so be warned! A good portfolio cannot be put together at the last minute. It is something that has be crafted over your career:

Be organized. If your portfolio looks like a dog's dinner it speaks volumes about your record-keeping and professional skills. Everything must be ordered and categorized in the right sections (see **CHAPTER 3, P.27** for more advice on an organized portfolio).

Record everything. It helps if you have an obsessive–compulsive streak. If it wasn't recorded, it didn't happen. If you did a procedure, record it in your logbook. If you presented at teaching, collect the feedback you received. If you attended a course or teaching, keep the certificate. Printouts of audits, presentations, and publications must be included.

Be reflective. Selectors like candidates who are able to reflect, as it suggests they can learn from past events. You should record reflective practice on your portfolio regularly. Try to record at least one session weekly. You can use any teaching, clinical event, or private study as an opportunity to reflect. If you have an e-portfolio, link it with a curriculum item.

Personal development plan. Every self-respecting portfolio should have one. Sit down and take the time to create one. Your goals should be specific with a clear timescale.

Work-based assessments. Aim to have significantly more assessments than the minimum. Try to spread them over a wide area of your curriculum.

Practical procedures

Document everything! As you progress through your career, keep a logbook of all the procedures and cases you have been involved with. Details to include are the date, the procedure name, patient ID, complications, findings or outcome, your role (first operator, second operator), if it was supervised, and, ideally, a signature from a witness.

Keep your e-portfolio updated with multiple Direct Observation of Procedural Skills (DOPS) assessments for each procedure. For specialties with practical procedures, the numbers of DOPS or cases are sometimes counted to allocate a short-listing score.

The best way to learn practical procedures is from an experienced operator. You must be forward and ask if they can teach you—stay silent and this chance may pass. Most seniors will be more than happy to teach you.

Courses

In addition to the mandatory resuscitation courses, attend other specialty-related courses. This demonstrates your interest in the specialty and could give you additional points at short-listing (up to a maximum of four or five courses in most cases). In **CHAPTER 7**, I list the courses which are relevant for each specialty. Many specialties also display their short-listing framework and check against this.

Management

Management experience in some specialties contributes towards your short-listing score, particularly at level ST3+. Take every opportunity to gain management experience throughout your career. This may include the following:

- Specialty training committee (trainee representative)
- Doctors' Mess committee member
- Club or society committee member

In addition, there are introductory courses to management and leadership skills organized by different companies. It is worth attending these if your specialty's short-list marking scheme take management qualifications into account.

REFERENCES

1 Dacre, J. *et al.* (2008). *Clinical problem solving test pilot.* Project Report. Royal College of Physicians, London (available at: www.ucl.ac.uk/dome/research/clinprob).

2 Jones, G. and Bunce, J. (2009). *Do you have to do a surgical F2 post to get a Core Training (CT1) in Surgery?* NHS South West, Peninsula Foundation School (available at: http://www.peninsuladeanery.nhs.uk/files/File/foundation/Feedback/Surgical_appointments_CT1_v9_230209.pdf).

CHAPTER 3

Being prepared

Applying for specialty training isn't simply about filling in an application form and popping in for an interview. When the time is right, you need to spring into action at short notice. To be able to do this, you need to be prepared—do your research, get your paperwork in order, and get equipped. You'll also have to monitor the situation regularly and keep your ear close to the ground.

Forewarned is forearmed

To do well, you need to know what the selection process entails. The deanery and royal college websites should be your first port of call. Find out as much as you can about the upcoming selection process. If you need more information, e-mail them directly. Be polite but persistent. If your e-mails go unanswered, telephone instead.

These are the questions you need answered:

- Is the application process national or local (individual deaneries)?
- If recruitment is national, which is the host deanery or organization?
- When is the application window expected to open (estimated dates will do)?
- When is the anticipated interview period?
- Is a selection exam anticipated?

Deaneries may not be able to reveal all the above information early on and it is worth contacting them again at a later date.

Applications: you snooze, you lose

In the past, some training posts were advertised for just a few days, with only a week before the application deadline. According to the MMC website (www.mmc.nhs.uk), deaneries need to advertise a job for only 3 days and can give you as few as 5 days to submit an application. Five days out of 365 days in a year! Unsurprisingly, many potential applicants will miss this tiny window of opportunity. No deanery will admit that this is intentional, but having a tiny application window in effect catches out those applicants who are unprepared (hence less motivated); a *de facto* form of short-listing!

You need to know when applications are expected to open. A couple of months before the anticipated application window, monitor the relevant deanery website(s) regularly. As a minimum do this weekly; twice weekly if you can. In addition to deanery websites, monitor the relevant royal college's website and NHS Jobs (www.jobs.nhs.uk). There may be last minute changes to application schedules and you might be given preliminary information on the application process such as selection exams.

Some websites such as NHS Jobs and BMJ Careers (careers.bmj.com) allow you to sign up for e-mail 'alerts' for posts fitting your criteria. Make use of this facility, but you should still visit deanery websites regularly.

Selection exams

Many specialties will roll out selection exams as part of their short-listing process in the coming years. Finding out about this in advance will give you a head start. As for any professional exam, start your revision early on. There are already many websites where you can practice questions for selection exams. Selection exams will be dealt with fully in **CHAPTER 4 (P47)**.

Interviews: you've got mail

After submitting your application form, check your e-mail inbox EVERY DAY. Invitations to interview are usually sent via e-mail. Sometimes, only 48 hours may be given for a response. Miss this e-mail and you could lose your interview place. Also, the sooner you respond, the more choice of interview slots you will have.

Find out the anticipated interview period. Knowing this will allow you to schedule your time. It's best to protect this period and be sure that you are available to respond. Do NOT book a holiday and do not undertake major commitments during this time if at all possible. Interviews are usually held over a few days. If you are out of the country or unavailable during this period, tough! Deaneries are on a tight schedule and you will get little sympathy.

Start your interview preparation months in advance (for more on interview preparation see **CHAPTERS 5 AND 6**).

Where to apply?

Is the application process organized nationally by a single 'host' deanery or is it organized locally by local deaneries? Knowing which could influence your application strategy. If it is a national process, you make a single application. Make sure you identify the host deanery; contact them, and monitor their website as described above.

If recruitment is local then you can apply to as many different deaneries as possible. The more deaneries you apply to, the better your chances of getting interviewed and the more shots you get at the pie. If you are not geographically restricted, seriously consider applying to as many deaneries as is practical. If you have a mortgage, remember that deaneries usually reimburse successful applicants for items such as estate agents' fees, removal fees, house-hunting trips, and stamp duty on newly bought properties.

Get kitted out

Virtually all applications for training posts are made online. This means that as a minimum you need access to a computer with an internet connection and a quiet place where you can work undisturbed. Ideally, this should be at home and NOT in the doctor's mess or hospital library as you will inadvertently be distracted by idle chatter with colleagues. (You can skip this section if you already have all of the above.)

For many professional reasons, you need to own your own computer. In addition to job applications, journals, educational resources, e-portfolios, and clinical guidelines are all online. A laptop is ideal because it is mobile. A basic laptop can be yours for under £300. You don't need a high-performance laptop unless you intend to play games or write computer programs.

You'll also need internet access, and a broadband connection is ideal. The simplest option is to get pay-as-you-go mobile broadband. All the major mobile networks provide this service; visit them online or pop into a store.

Owning an all-in-one printer (with scanner) isn't essential, but is very convenient when you are organizing your paper portfolio. It lets you scan, print, and copy documents at home, saving you trips to the library. Plus, printing personal material at work is actually illegal. A basic model costs £40 and I recommend getting one if you are not financially stretched.

Preparing your portfolio

Organizing your portfolio can be a time-consuming process. Getting it sorted out beforehand allows you to focus on applications and interviews when the time comes. Most specialties now have a portfolio station which accounts for a significant proportion of your interview score. The presentation and organization of your portfolio will be judged. Also, organizing your portfolio will refresh your memory and give you new ideas for your application form. For a first class portfolio:

- Gather your certificates for degrees, diplomas, prizes, and courses. Print out all your assessments, appraisals, publications, audits, presentations, and teaching slides. Include correspondence such as e-mails on pending publications, MDs, or PhDs. Feedback from presentations or teaching should also be here. Don't forget any 'thank you' cards and letters of praise from patients or colleagues.

- Buy a large, good quality ring binder, preferably in a dark colour with about 10 dividers. The dividers must have tabs on the side that stick out. You will also need approximately 200 clear A4 pockets (avoid the cheap flimsy ones). Buy good quality materials.

- Use the dividers to separate your folder into different sections. I suggest the following: qualifications, prizes, publications, DOPs, other assessments (i.e. CEX, CBD, MSF), audits, research, presentations, teaching, others. You can devise your own method of organization.

- Customize your portfolio to show off your strengths; for example if you have lots of publications, position this section near the front.

- For every clear pocket, there should only be two sheets of paper arranged back-to-back. Your portfolio can be read by turning the clear pockets without taking any sheets out.

- Organize each section chronologically with the most recent documents towards the front. For each section, create a summary page, listing all the contents. This summary page should be printed out on one side in a large font for easy reading.

- At the front of your portfolio, create a contents page. Physically align the heading for each section with the appropriate divider tab. It might be easier to do this by hand, but write neatly! Another way is to label each tab. Evaluators can go through your portfolio quickly and don't have to struggle through it.

- Just behind your contents page, include an up-to-date copy of your CV or your application form. Although not essential, it makes it easier for the assessor to view your career as a whole.

In **CHAPTER 5** there will be more advice on the portfolio station at interview.

Reflective practice

If you encounter an event which serves as a learning point, make a record of it and the lessons you have learnt. Note down how you have changed your practice as a result of it. This could be a clinical event, teaching, or a discussion with your seniors. Keeping a log of such events in your portfolio will serve as evidence of your ability to reflect, a desirable criterion in many specialties. Evidence of reflective practice may be noted at portfolio stations.

More importantly, your log of events will serve as a useful *aide-mémoire* when it comes to application forms and interviews. Many questions that you are asked will be based around your past behaviour. Examples of such questions are:

- Describe a mistake you made professionally and how you managed it.
- When did you last disagree with a colleague and how did you deal with it?
- Describe a scenario in which you played an important role as part of a team.

It is hard to recall such events if you are put on the spot, and the details often fade with time. As I'll elaborate further in **CHAPTER 5**, the scenario that you use will influence how well you'll do at selection. A log of such events will mean you can draw on a larger selection of events and hopefully choose the most appropriate one.

Essential paperwork

You have to sort this out now. When you get an invitation to interview, you will want to concentrate on preparing for the interview and not stressing out on tedious paperwork.

Alert your referees. Approach them and ask if they would be willing to provide references. If it was over a year since you worked with them, you will need to subtly jog their memory. Provide them with the dates you worked for them, on which ward, and in what capacity. Remember, consultants are busy people and there may be a delay before you get a response—a telephone reminder via their secretaries will help.

Have other essential documents together in a folder. These should include your health records, immunization record, recent payslips, and your CRB (Criminal Records Bureau) check. If you are British or a citizen of another EU country you need to bring a copy of your passport and/or birth certificate. Non-EU citizens should bring their passport and a Home Office letter stipulating their entitlement to work in the UK. If applicable, bring your IELTS (International English Language Testing System) certificate.

Often you have to provide proofs of your address, such as utility bills and bank statements. You may be required to bring proof of foundation competencies. This is either a sign-off from your foundation years or proof of working in educationally approved SHO (senior house officer) posts.

Make photocopies of everything described above. Deaneries usually ask you to bring photocopies and will want to hold on to these for their records. Making copies in advance saves you a lot of hassle. Last but not least, have two passport photos ready for each interview. Remember to dress professionally for the photo.

CHAPTER 4

The application form

Introduction

A well-completed application form is the first step on your journey to specialty training. However, filling forms in can be a real pain; believe me, I've filled in more than I care to remember!

Deaneries score each eligible application form they receive using a protocol. Only applicants with the highest scores get short-listed for interview. At interview, applicants are again scored based on their performance on the day. The short-list score and the interview score are added up to give a final score. The applicants with the highest final scores will be offered a job. An applicant's short-list score accounts for about 20% to 40% of an applicant's final score.

> Application form score
> +
> Interview score =
> Job offer (if the total is enough)

The application form is your chance to sell yourself. In this chapter, I will reveal precisely how deaneries score applicants and provide suggestions on how to maximize your short-list score.

Get the short-list protocol

Search the recruiting deanery's website for the short-list protocol. If it is not on their website, contact the deanery directly. Be polite but persistent; if your e-mail is ignored, telephone the deanery. They may release the short-list protocol only on request. Unfortunately, the protocol is not always released to applicants—despite the MMC website stating *'Details of the short-listing and interview scoring scheme should be made available to you on request.'*

The essence of 100 short-listing protocols

The advice in this chapter is based on my research of over a hundred short-listing protocols from 11 deaneries and several royal societies. All the short-listing protocols I have read are in the public domain, but finding some has required hours of searching. I have researched as many specialties as I could find.

I can't tell you **exactly** how each deanery will short-list applicants. Each short-listing protocol is slightly different. But regardless of deanery and specialty, most protocols score applicants along remarkably similar lines. I have taken these protocols and condensed them into this chapter.

Read the application form and instructions

Before you answer a single question on the application form, read it and any accompanying instructions carefully. The designers of application forms usually try to guide applicants to give their best responses, and there are often clues to help you. Answer the question precisely and in the format that has been requested.

Let me illustrate with a sample question from the application form for Core Medical Training (2009) designed by the Royal College of Physicians, London:

> In this section please provide details of clinical audit experience, giving titles and dates. What specifically was your contribution, what did the audit show, was the audit presented or published and was the audit cycle closed?

These two sentences ask for lots of details: *'What specifically was your contribution…'*. Short-list protocols award points if the applicant has initiated, designed, or lead an audit. Further, *'…was the audit presented or published and was the audit cycle closed?'*: again, most short-list protocols award additional points if the audit was presented, published, or re-audited. Applicants who ignore the above instructions and list the audits they have participated in without elaborating further will deprive themselves of valuable short-list points.

Presentation matters

Your application form represents you; it should be well-presented. You wouldn't dream of turning up to a job interview in a grubby T-shirt and a pair of tatty jeans! Submitting a poorly presented application form is just as bad. If you present your responses well it is easier to score your application form correctly, and it is less likely that crucial information will be missed.

Proof-read your application form for spelling or grammatical errors, correct punctuation, and capitalization. You can run a spell check by copying your answer from the application form into Microsoft Word. However, there is no replacement for a thorough proof-reading. Try not to proof-read your responses straight away. Review it with fresh eyes a few hours later or even the next day if you can. Mistakes will be easier to spot.

Unless the application form specifies otherwise, consider using bullet points in parts of the application form. It is easier to read and looks neater. Bullet points are particularly handy for lists such as publications, prizes, and audits.

Clear and concise English

Expressing yourself well on paper reflects on your ability to communicate, so make the effort to complete your application form in well-written English. I am not suggesting you should write like Shakespeare. Rather, your writing should be concise and easy to understand. Use the correct grammar and avoid basic mistakes. **Some short-listing protocols mark the clarity of your English:** this mark accounts for approximately 8% of the short-list score.

Writing well is a skill that takes time to develop. But here are a few golden rules to follow to help you to improve your writing:

- Be concise and avoid waffling. You will have a word limit; every word must 'work' towards selling you. If a word or phrase is redundant, omit it. It is a common error to use certain phrases in an attempt to sound intelligent. Examples of such waffle are: 'as a matter of fact', 'basically', 'last but not least', 'at this moment in time', 'obviously' (if it's so obvious, why say so), 'on the basis of', 'except for the fact that'.

- Use plain English, not gobbledegook! Instead of the phrase 'health-care professional', use doctor or nurse. 'Hospital occupancy administrator' can be replaced by 'bed manager'. A 'physical impairment aid' is better rephrased as a walking stick.

- Avoid long sentences; they make information harder to absorb and require greater concentration to follow.

- Keep your paragraphs short. Big blocks of text are a struggle to read and are a strain on the eyes. Faced with a giant block of text, an assessor may be tempted to skim read a paragraph, missing out vital information.

- The first sentences should convey the main point of each paragraph. The rest of the paragraph should then build upon the opening sentence. Each paragraph should pertain to the same topic. Newspapers use this technique with good effect.

- Use the active voice instead of the passive voice if you can. It sounds more personal and interesting. Medical literature encourages use of the passive voice. Resist the urge! Which of the two paragraphs below is easier to read?

Passive voice: The idea of an audit of our antibiotic usage was initiated by myself and was proposed to my consultant. My idea was enthusiastically received.

Active voice: It was initially my idea to audit our antibiotic usage and I proposed this to my consultant. He received my idea enthusiastically.

For further information on how to improve your writing, I recommend a short book, *Improve your Writing Skills* by Graham King (Collins, 2009).

Copy and paste with care

Isn't technology wonderful? You can 'copy' your answers from an old application form and 'paste' them into a different one. Be careful! Even if the question on the application form is the same, the instructions may be different. You may also need to reformat the answer if the word limit is different. Your circumstances may have changed and an up-to-date answer would be more appropriate.

If you are applying to a different grade or specialty, then take extra care. Make sure the answer you give is still appropriate. Perhaps a more specialty-specific answer would be better.

Don't be late like Cinderella

It's blindingly obvious isn't it? Who could be so daft as to submit an application late! So why, in 2008, did over 400 doctors miss the North West Deanery's application deadline?[1] Few doctors would intentionally make such a mistake. Too many of them left their application form to almost the last minute: 54% of doctors submitted their applications on the last day and most of these applications were submitted just 15 minutes before the deadline.[1] Don't get caught out; otherwise, like Cinderella, your golden carriage to specialty training will disappear before your eyes!

Why take such a high-risk approach? Anything could happen on the last day or last hour. Your computer could freeze, your internet connection might fail, you could fall ill, or the deanery's server could crash under the deluge. Aim to submit your application a few days before the deadline and stick to it.

Crafting a good application takes time, often a lot more than you think! As a minimum, allocate yourself a couple of hours over a week. Set yourself targets for each day. For example: Monday, prizes and audits; Tuesday, research and publications; Wednesday, teaching, commitment to specialty. Always give yourself a few extra days in reserve—life is unpredictable, be realistic.

> Submit your application form a few days early.
> Don't get caught out!

Essential criteria

First things first: check that you fulfil **all** the essential criteria. Your medical degree, eligibility for GMC registration, Foundation competencies, and immigration status fall under this category. If you don't fulfil all the essential criteria, you won't be considered any further—so don't waste your energy. If you are in this situation, now is the time to reconsider your options: apply for a different post or work towards rectifying the situation.

Additional undergraduate degrees

The majority of short-listing protocols will award points if you hold an additional undergraduate degree such as a BSc, BA, BMedSci, or equivalent. If you were awarded a 1st class degree or a 2:1, state this clearly as you will get more points. State whether your degree was intercalated, as additional points are awarded for this by some deaneries.

Sample response

Degree	Class	Date	Awarding body
BSc (intercalated)	2:1	June 2005	University of London

Sample scoring protocol

Degree	Points (max. 8)
Intercalated BA or BSc 1st class	8
Intercalated BA or BSc 2:1	6
Undergraduate degree before medicine 1st class	6
Intercalated BA or BSc 2:2	4
Intercalated BA or BSc other	2
Undergraduate degree before medicine 2:1	2

Postgraduate degrees and diplomas

PhD, MD, MPhil, or MSc degrees all will attract points. If your PhD or MSc was based on original research (defending a thesis) state this as it will attract more points. You should also write down any other postgraduate diplomas in this section, even if they relate to a different specialty. Examples of diplomas include DRCOG, DCH, FFP, and DGO.

If you are undertaking a postgraduate degree but it has not yet been awarded, mention it anyway. Describe what stage you are at, i.e. registered, in preparation, submitted, awaiting viva. Some short-listing protocols will award points for degrees that are in progress. It is certainly worth a try and doesn't hurt provided you state that the degree has not yet been awarded.

Suggested response

Postgraduate degree	Date	Awarding body
MSc (original research thesis)	July 2004	Cardiff University
PhD (bound and submitted)	Not yet awarded	Bristol University

Sample scoring protocol (ST3, Trauma, and Orthopaedics)

Postgraduate degree	Points (max. 8)
PhD by thesis	8
MD (original research)	6
MPhil, MD (dissertation)	4
MSc or PhD in progress	3
Other diploma or MD in progress	2

Royal college examinations

List all royal college examinations you have passed even if they were in a different specialty. They may still be relevant and get you points. For example, MRCS and MRCP may both be applicable for Radiology, Emergency Medicine, and Obstetrics and Gynaecology. If you have passed only part of the full exam, i.e. FRCA MCQ exam,

MRCPCH Part 1a, MRCS Part 1, you should still include this. A pass in part of an exam will attract points.

Include the date you passed the exam. A few short-listing protocols award additional points if you achieved full membership quickly, i.e. within 3 years of graduation. Sometimes, you are required to list your royal college exams in the postgraduate degree section.

Sample scoring protocol (ST2, Paediatrics)

Exam	Points
MRCPCH Parts 1a and 1b	4
MRCPCH Part 1a	2

Training courses

List the resuscitation courses you have completed such as ALS, ILS, APLS, ATLS, APLS, or ALERT. If you were identified as having instructor potential, highlight this. You can include other courses such as relevant seminars, conferences, practical skills, teaching, and critical appraisal. Don't leave this section blank, and search your memory hard for relevant courses.

Courses that are relevant to the specialty attract more points. In **CHAPTER 7**, I list courses that are relevant for each specialty.

Sample scoring protocol (CT1, Surgery)

Course	Points (max. 3)
Attended more than one course relevant to specialty	3
Attended one course relevant to specialty	2
Attended course/s unrelated to specialty	1
No evidence of courses attended	0

Relevant courses include Basic Surgical Skills, ATLS, CCrISP, ALS, APLS, and Royal College of Surgeons courses.

Prizes

Don't worry if you find this section a struggle, you're in good company. Scour your memory banks and medical school folders thoroughly for awards. You can include bursaries, scholarships; merits or distinctions awarded for a module or term; essay prizes, or any other awards. Runner-up prizes or bronze medals still count. Only awards in higher education will be considered, so don't be tempted to include prizes from school days (unless they were particularly prestigious, e.g. national or international awards).

Distinctions or honours awarded as part of a degree (MBBS or BSc) tend to attract more points. So do national and international prizes. If you have such an award, state this clearly on your application form. Don't assume that everybody knows the significance of your award.

How you describe your prize can affect your score. Below is a sample response from John, a fictional ST2 applicant to Core Medical Training. Use the sample short-listing protocol below to score John's response.

John's application form—prize section

- November 2007—AC Comfort Prize; prize for essay entitled 'Technology and its effects on ageing in the 21st century'.
- June 2002—Educational bursary awarded a sum of £1500.

Sample short-listing protocol

Prize	Points (max. 5 points)
International or national prize	4
Prize awarded as part of final MB	3
Prize awarded as part of undergraduate course	1
Scholarships or bursaries for medical school	1
Other undergraduate or postgraduate prizes	1

How many points did you award John? Two points in total? Was John's bursary awarded for medical school? It isn't clear what kind of prize he was awarded. If you were an assessor with hundreds of application forms to evaluate that day, would you take the trouble to find out what sort of prize John was awarded? I have rewritten John's answer below. Try and rescore John's application.

Revised version of John's application form—prize section

- **November 2007—national prize (AC Comfort Prize) awarded by the Royal Society of Medicine** for essay entitled 'Technology and its effects on ageing in the 21st century', published in the *Journal of the Royal Society of Medicine*, December 2007.
- **June 2002—bursary of £1500 awarded by UCL School of Medicine** to pursue undergraduate training. Only 5 students out of 300 were awarded this bursary in 2002.

Emphasize the word 'national'. Words near the top and upper left-hand corner of any paragraph attract the most attention. Displaying the words in bold accentuates this. Adding details like where your prize was presented or the amount of funds awarded in your bursary gives it a final flourish. How many applicants were awarded your prize? Sure, it is shameless self-promotion, but this is what you need to do to stand out. The revised version of John's application form would achieve the maximum score of five points.

Publications

Don't despair if you don't have a peer-reviewed paper to your name. Unless specified otherwise (on the application form) you can include other types of publications, for example letters to the editor, articles in newspapers and magazines, book contributions, patient advisory leaflets, newsletters, online articles. Leaving this section blank will guarantee zero points and will not impress at interview. By including other publication types at least you stand a chance of earning points, depending on the short-list protocol and discretion of the assessors. Getting a peer-reviewed publication is not as hard as you might think—read **CHAPTER 2** for advice on getting published.

Some short-listing protocols award points for online contributions. Have you ever made an electronic comment on an online publication? For example, BMJ.com allows readers to post a 'rapid response'.

If you have a string of peer-reviewed papers to your name, list them chronologically with the most recent first. Utilize the 'bold' function to highlight publications that are relevant to the specialty or are in a prestigious journal so that there is no chance they are missed. Again, this is shameless self-promotion, but isn't that what your application form is for?

Include papers that have been accepted for publication but not yet out in print. This is perfectly legitimate provided you state this on the application form. Make sure you bring evidence of acceptance to your interview (e.g. an e-mail from the editor).

Presentations

List all the presentations you have made, in chronological order. You can include presentations at audit meetings, grand rounds, departmental meetings, poster presentations, journal club, and teaching sessions. Try to list about five presentations. You will usually get a point for each presentation, up to a maximum score of 4 or 5. If you've presented more times than this, be selective:

- Always include international, national, or regional presentations as these score the most points. It doesn't matter if the presentation was in a different specialty
- Choose presentations that are relevant to the specialty.

If you've presented at an international, national, or regional meeting then make this clear on your form. Not everybody will know what type of meeting you presented at just by the name. To illustrate, can you work out if the presentation below was at a local or regional meeting?

- John Radcliffe Hospital, grand round, April 2009: case presentation of an intravenous drug user with a femoral artery aneurysm.

It is difficult to be certain. The person doing the short-listing might be under a lot of pressure. He or she certainly won't spend hours agonizing over it! Make their lives easier and state the type of presentation clearly.

Below, I have rewritten the same presentation differently:

- **Regional grand round (Oxford Deanery)**, April 2009, John Radcliffe Hospital. Case presentation of an intravenous drug user with a femoral artery aneurysm.

Sample scoring protocol

Presentation type	Score (max. 5)
Presented at an international meeting	4
Presented at a national meeting	3
Presented at a regional meeting	2
Local presentation or poster	1

The key word is 'regional'. Writing it in bold and near the beginning emphasizes it. There is no official definition of a regional meeting. Broadly speaking, the audiences in regional meetings originate from across the county or deanery. Most of your audience will be employed by a few different NHS trusts. If your meeting fulfils the above criteria, it is safe to assume it was regional. Examples of regional meetings include deanery grand rounds, royal college regional gatherings, and county-wide specialty meetings.

Audit

As far as audits are concerned, quality is more important than quantity, so don't simply list all the audits you have participated in. Give as much detail as you can about each audit as it will improve your short-list score.

Below is the detail you should include for each audit:

- Who initiated or designed it. If you suggested the audit or played a role in designing it, say so!
- Who led it? If you were coordinating it, then it's fair to say you led it (under your consultant's supervision).
- Describe what you were auditing and the findings of your audit.
- Describe the recommendations you made. Were there any changes made as a result of your audit?
- Who were the findings presented to? What type of meeting was this?
- Were the findings published anywhere, e.g. hospital newsletter, website, or journal?
- Did you complete the audit cycle with a re-audit?

Most trainees change jobs frequently, making it impractical to undertake a 'hands-on' re-audit. But if you provided assistance or followed up the outcome of a re-audit then do mention it. If there was no re-audit or no chance to assist, you can still demonstrate in your response that you understand the importance of re-auditing and made steps to follow it up or offer assistance.

Most of the short-listing protocols I have read score the section on audits similarly. This is regardless of specialty or seniority. In general, points are awarded if the audit was:

- self-initiated
- self-designed
- led by the applicant
- presented at a meeting (additional points if national or regional)
- had recommendations or changes made as a result of it
- a re-audit or an attempt to follow up.

A few short-listing schemes also gave additional points if the audit was related to the specialty applied for.

Teaching

Most doctors have taught medical students or fellow doctors from time to time. So what is it that will really make you stand out? If you have taught using a variety of methods, e.g. lectures, small group teaching, or one-to-one sessions, then mention this. If you have received feedback in the form of an evaluation sheet or questionnaire, then state this. It is even better if have you received formal training or attended a course on teaching. If you teach on a regular basis then describe who you teach and the frequency of the sessions. Unless specified otherwise, you don't have to restrict yourself to medical teaching, for example do you coach a sport, teach religious lessons, or do other voluntary work of this type?

Sample scoring protocol

Teaching	Score (max. 5)
Have designed or led a regional/national teaching programme	4
Have designed or led a local teaching programme	3
Have formal training or have attended a course in teaching	2
Have a formal role or a regular slot in a teaching programme	2
Have formal feedback on teaching	2
Have taught using a variety of methods	1

Clinical and practical skills relevant to the specialty

In this section describe the skills you posses that are relevant to the specialty. You could describe your skills in bullet point form. Below are a few suggestions of what to include under this section:

- Clinical experience in the specialty: elaborate on the number of months and at what grade. Also elaborate further on your duties and the level of supervision required, i.e. outpatient clinics, inpatient care, elective procedures, reviewing inpatient referrals.
- Include clinical experience in other specialties if relevant. For example, if you are applying for Emergency Medicine, experience in Medicine, Surgery, Radiology, and Intensive Care would be helpful. Explain how your experience in other areas is relevant.
- Highlight any unique experience. For example, have you worked in a tertiary centre or are skilled in a procedure not normally expected for your grade.
- Experience of on-call duty (unselected take). Again, describe the number of months and the grade.

- Practical skills and procedures that you have performed or assisted in. Describe the level of competency that you have achieved with each procedure, i.e. independent, under minimal supervision, second operator. It is even better if you can provide evidence in the form of DOPs or a logbook. If applying for a surgical specialty, elaborate on the number of procedures you have done or assisted with.
- Any training courses that you have attended, relevant to the specialty. Particularly impressive are courses that are not mandatory and require extra effort.

Commitment to the specialty

This is your chance to show that you eat, sleep, and breathe the specialty. Many short-listing protocols allocate a large chunk of the points to this section so it's worth spending a decent amount of time working on it. Your response must address two questions:

1. Why do you love this specialty?

Your reasons must be personal and include lots of details to give your response credibility. Reasons you could give include:

- inspiration from a particular person or doctor,
- motivation from a loved one's illness,
- enjoyment of the specialty as a medical student
- the practical procedures involved
- interest in the academic aspect of the specialty
- work–life balance
- anything else that is personal to you.

Select no more than three reasons and elaborate futher in detail. Whatever reasons you give, your enthusiasm must come across on paper. If you have time, leave your response aside and read it back to yourself a few days later. Imagine if you were the consultant. Are the words you have written believable? Is the explanation good and does the logic flow?

2. What did you do to find out more about the specialty? Show us how you have immersed yourself in it

On a piece of paper write what you have done to learn about the specialty. Let your mind flow and record anything that comes to mind. Here are examples of what you could include: electives, special study modules (SSMs), taster weeks, courses, talking to registrars and consultants, attending outpatients, observing procedures, scrubbing up in theatre, audits. When writing your response you can choose what you wish to include from this list. Include details such as date, hospital, and consultant to give your response credibility. It is important to describe what you have learnt from your experiences.

Below is a sample response for an ST1 applicant in Neurosurgery. Note the details and the lessons learnt.

> In my final year of medical school I applied for rotations that included neurosurgery. In my 4 month Foundation Year post with Mr Brain at Charing Cross Hospital (London) I had the opportunity to 'scrub-up' in theatre. Observing first-hand, I realised how much mental and physical stamina was required. I also observed over a dozen neurosurgical clinics. There, I had the opportunity to discuss the pros and cons of the specialty with neurosurgeons and trainees alike. Despite the many extra years of training required, a career in neurosurgery sounds extremely rewarding.

If you have worked in the specialty, what grade was it and for how long? Describe specific roles like attending outpatients, reviewing referrals, caring for inpatients, consenting patients for procedures, etc. Were there any specialty-related skills you learnt from the post? Did you complete any exams or attend courses and conferences? Include related audits, presentations, prizes, and publications. If you invested a significant amount of time and effort like a research project, PhD, or MD this will be particularly impressive.

Personal statement

You may be asked to give a personal statement. **Read the instructions carefully and follow them!** The response that is expected varies with each application form. You may be asked to elaborate on any of the following areas:

- commitment to specialty
- clinical and practical skills
- why you have chosen this specialty.

You may also be asked to give information that has not been covered in the other questions. If this is the case, methodically go through the person specifications and identify the remaining areas. Don't throw away points and don't leave this section empty.

Achievements and extracurricular activities

To ace this question, you need to:

- demonstrate significant achievements
- relate your achievements to the specialty you are applying for.

The significance of your achievements with be judged. Choose outstanding ones such as those at international or national level, those requiring above average talent, or those that require a significant amount of effort or sacrifice.

Don't worry if you aren't an X-Factor or Wimbledon finalist! Even relatively modest achievements can be written up in a positive light. This is not the time for understatement; don't be ashamed to do some self-promotion. Emphasize how much effort was required to achieve your goal. For example, if you completed a marathon, you can explain that it required several months of training, running an average of 40 miles a week. Your ability to stick to your training schedule proves your dedication, motivation, and ability to plan for the long term.

Your achievement must make you look good. Don't include achievements that most junior doctors have such as a driving licence, Basic Life Support, or secondary school prizes. If your achievement is related to medicine but outside of the medical school course or NHS work, you could still include it here. Examples include research, teaching doctors, and presenting at conferences.

For example, if you enjoy scuba diving abroad and are certified, you could say:

I am a certified PADI Open Water Diver. This is an internationally recognized qualification requiring satisfactory theory and practical assessments, followed by a minimum number of dives in open water. I enjoy the challenge of diving in different locations like Egypt, Malaysia, and the Maldives. I believe in the need for continuous self-improvement and am working towards PADI Advanced Diver certification.

Whatever your achievement, it is important to link it your specialty. This is just as important as the significance of your achievement. For example, if you are an accomplished musician, this can demonstrate discipline, dedication, or manual dexterity:

I am an accomplished pianist, having completed Grade 8 by the age of 17. I have played for my university orchestra, performing at a variety of venues including the Royal Albert Hall, Budapest Opera House, and St Paul's Cathedral. To achieve such a level of competence requires steadfast dedication and thousands of hours of practice. Likewise, training to become a skilled surgeon requires the same demonstration of dedication and tenacity. My piano skills also demonstrate my manual dexterity and finger coordination; a necessity for any surgeon.

Below is a list of achievements accompanied by attributes that these could demonstrate:

- Accomplished sportsperson: stamina, dedication, coordination, focus
- Event organizer: organization, leadership, initiative
- Group leader/committee member: leadership, keen teacher, management skills
- Fundraising for charity: caring, determination, initiative

- Completing a marathon: long-term planning, dedication, motivation
- Politics: leadership, communication skills
- Acting (theatre): creativity, communication skills, dedication
- Writing, journalism, blogging: creativity, inquisitiveness, communication skills
- Website and computing: learning new skills, competent with technology
- Certified scuba diver: planning, concentration, focus

Leadership and teamwork

Read the application form carefully. Is it asking you to **list** examples of your teamwork and/or leadership roles? Or is it asking for you to **describe** a scenario in which you were leader or part of a team?

If you need to describe a scenario where you were a team player, choose an example that involved a variety of professionals, e.g. physiotherapist, social workers, district nurses. Your response must focus on your role as much as possible. Give details of how you communicated, negotiated, or cooperated with other teams. Use 'I' instead of 'we'. Explain your contribution and demonstrate how your involvement affected the outcome. If you are asked to list leadership roles, then there is some overlap with the section on Management below.

Management

Questions about your management experience tend to appear at ST3+. Try not to leave this section blank. The chances are that you have held a position of responsibility before. As a junior doctor, consider positions such as BMA or Remedy UK representative, on-call rota organizer, teaching organizer, doctors' mess committee, specialty training committee representative, etc. Go through your medical school years and think of all the sports, societies, unions, and clubs you were involved in. Management experience outside of medicine could count, so consider including businesses, charities, and clubs that you are involved in.

Management at national or regional level will attract a higher score. If the committee you sat on was national, regional, or deanery-wide then state this clearly. Use the 'bold' function on the relevant keyword. A management qualification or diploma might be awarded a higher score; such as an intercalated BSc in management.

Information technology (IT)

Most application forms don't ask about IT skills. There are still a few exceptions and for this reason I have included a few lines of advice. If you are asked about your IT skills, describe which applications you are competent in; internet browsing, e-mail, word processing, PowerPoint presentations, spreadsheets, databases, statistical software. Mention if you have completed an IT course (e.g. European Computer Driving Licence) and bring your certificates to interview. For full marks you need to demonstrate more advanced skills like website or database design, knowledge of a programming language (e.g. C++, HTML). If you think a mouse is a small furry animal you need to work on your IT skills (see **CHAPTER 2** on career development).

Sample scoring protocol

IT skill	Score (max. 3)
Design of national database or website	3
Design of local database or website	2
Basic IT skills, i.e. word processing, internet	1

Selection exams

At the time of writing (2010), only applicants to General Practice and Public Health had to sit exams. It is likely that other specialties, particularly for CT1/ST1, will incorporate exams in the future. Anaesthesia, ACCS, Psychiatry, Paediatrics, CMT, and Surgery have piloted selection exams. The results suggest that selection exams are better than application forms at predicting an applicant's interview performance. Another plus is that exams can be computer-marked, making them cheaper and more time-efficient. It looks like exams are here to stay! There are two main types of selection exams being piloted:

- clinical knowledge tests
- situational judgement tests (professional dilemmas).

As in any exam, preparation is essential for a good score. Start your revision a few months in advance, particularly if applying to a competitive specialty. If you don't, your competitors will.

Exam strategy

- Read the instructions before you start the exam. Instructions can change from year to year. Pay attention to how many questions and pages there should be and check this before you start.

- Read the entire question carefully before you answer. The presence of a single word can change everything.
- Pay particular attention to the last sentence of the question. For example, 'what is the next test you should organize?' can be completely different from 'what is the most diagnostic test?'.
- Do not select a response until you have read all the possible options.
- Often, the correct response will not be obvious and you must make your best guess. Improve your odds by eliminating the options that are likely to be wrong.
- If there is no negative marking, you should always select an answer, even if it is a pure guess. At least you stand a chance of earning points. Leave it empty and you are guaranteed nothing.
- If you have to guess, remember that there are very few absolutes in medicine. An option containing 'always' or 'never' is more likely to be false. An option containing 'may' or 'could' is more likely to be true.

Time it right

- Many applicants run out of time during an exam. Pace yourself and set targets in advance. I recommend, 25%, 50%, and 75% targets. For example, if you have a 1-hour exam with 40 questions, I suggest a target of 10 questions at 15 minutes, 20 questions at 30 minutes, and 30 questions at 45 minutes.
- Be strict with your targets. If you fall behind, speed up, even if you have to start making guesses.
- Closer to exam day, practice with a few mock exams under timed conditions.

The clinical problem solving test

As the name suggests, this is a clinical knowledge test, usually in the form of an EMQ (extended matching question) or SBA (single-best answer). ST1 applicants will be tested at Foundation level and it will be on investigation, diagnosis, or management of a condition.

> Practice questions over and over again!

- Practice as many questions as you can. This is the most time-efficient method. Many applicants practice over a thousand questions from many books and/or websites. Reattempt the questions you have a made mistake in at a later date.

- Good revision books and/or websites are not cheap but if they help you get the career of your dreams it represents a worthwhile investment. Names such as EMedica, ISC Medical, Onexamination, and Pastest have been recommended by previous applicants.
- Learn from your mistakes in practice questions. Read the accompanying explanations and try to learn from them. Look the answer up in a book if you have to. Make a quick note of what you have learnt: this will aid your revision.
- Prepare for the right level. If applying for ST1, the exam will be at the level of FY1–2. Use concise books such as the *Oxford Handbook of Clinical Medicine* and the *Oxford Handbook of Specialties* for reference. The bigger the book, the less likely you will read it.
- Do **not** read your reference books from cover to cover. Instead, I recommend dipping into them when required, i.e. when you make a mistake or are weak in a particular area.
- Revision improves recall. Reattempt the questions you have made mistakes in and regularly review the notes you have made.
- Spread your revision and cover broad areas. Do not focus heavily on a particular specialty. The exam is meant to be very broad. The exam piloted by the Academy of Medical Colleges in 2010 contained questions in Medicine, Surgery, Psychiatry, Pharmacology, and Paediatrics.
- For ST1 entry, the level of knowledge required will be at Foundation level.

The situational judgement test (SJT)

This is a written psychometric test. Each question has a professional dilemma with a list of possible responses. Applicants have to rank the responses in order of 'appropriateness'. Those who rank their responses similarly to senior doctors in the specialty will score the highest.

Familiarize yourself with the GMC's Good Medical Practice (www.gmc-uk.org/guidance/good_medical_practice.asp). This forms the basis of the marking scheme. Guidance that uses the word 'must' is an overriding principle and **always** has to be adhered to. Guidance with the word 'should' will apply in **most** circumstances (there are exceptions).

Practice as many questions as possible. There are many websites and books you can use. Practice questions will teach you the 'correct' responses. SJTs are meant to be psychometric tests and not knowledge based. Nevertheless, there is evidence that practice can improve your scores. Read all the possible responses before answering. Often, the best and worst responses will be easiest to spot. You can then rank the remaining responses.

Below are a few guiding principles that I have distilled:

- Patient safety and care is always your first priority. If patient safety is at risk, you must act to remove and report it.
- If you have to choose, treat the sickest patients first. Treat the patient who is likely to die soonest (unless they are not for resuscitation).
- If you have to choose between two equally sick patients, your first duty of care is to the patient in front of you. Ask for help or give telephone advice for the second patient. Leave only when the first patient is stable.
- Lying or fraudulent behaviour is an absolute no.
- Patient confidentiality is to be respected, with very few exceptions (i.e. someone is at risk of serious harm or terrorist threat).
- Blaming colleagues is unprofessional.
- Do not put your personal safety at risk. This ultimately affects patient care.
- If you are inexperienced or do not know what you are doing, stop and seek help. Do not proceed alone even if your consultant insists (patient safety).
- Ignoring a problem or just leaving it to somebody else is usually a bad idea.
- In general, asking for help or involving seniors is a good idea.
- If you have a problem with a colleague, talking to them first is usually the best course of action.
- If a mistake has been made, tell the patient and apologise as soon as you can. Rectify it if possible. It doesn't matter if the mistake was not your fault.
- If there are multiple issues requiring attention, categorize them into three groups: emergency (now!), urgent (very soon), routine (when convenient).

In summary

- Fill in your application form as well as you can; it is your ticket to getting a training job.
- Get your hands on the short-list protocol.
- Follow the instructions on the application form; they are there to help.
- Answer the application form concisely without unnecessary words.
- List all the parts of postgraduate exams that you have passed.
- For prizes describe how many applicants you beat to win your prize. Emphasize if the prize was national or international.

- Describe your role in audits precisely and try to describe a re-audit if possible.
- For teaching emphasize any feedback or formal roles you have had.
- Consider publications other than peer-reviewed ones.
- Demonstrate commitment to specialty—show how you eat, drink, and sleep the specialty!
- You must prepare for selection exams as you would for any other exam.

REFERENCE

1 *Quick Guide to recruitment in 2010*. Department of Health Modernising Medical Careers Programme Team. www.mmc.nhs.uk

CHAPTER 5

Interview and assessment stations: how to excel

Introduction

The word 'interview' strikes fear into the mind of some doctors; it shouldn't if you are prepared. If you have recently been invited to interview, congratulations! You are at the final hurdle before the 'golden' training post. Don't celebrate just yet, there is still much to do. Jump straight to the 'Emergency interview schedule' (PAGE 59). If your interview is not imminent, carry on reading below.

Structured interview

The traditional interview has now been 'reincarnated' as the structured interview. Each interview usually lasts about 10 minutes, typically with two or three interviewers. For the purposes of this book, 'interview' will refer solely to structured interviews.

Each interviewer takes turns to question the applicant on a particular area, e.g. research, audit, teaching. After that, a different interviewer will take over the questioning, usually with a change in topic. The members of the panel who are not questioning will be busy listening and 'scoring' your performance. The idea is that each applicant will be scored independently by multiple interviewers on a variety of areas.

Most applicants to specialty training (excluding GP applicants) will encounter a structured interview as part of the selection process. Most selection centres will have at least one 'station' with a structured interview.

At more senior levels (ST3+) and for smaller specialties, structured interviews are still being used as the sole means of assessing candidates. If you are applying for a LAT post (locum appointment for training) this is also the most likely format.

Selection centre: interview and practical assessment

Don't be intimidated by the term 'selection centre'. It usually involves a selection process in which a combination of interviews and practical assessments are used. Candidates are assessed at multiple stations, moving around them at regular intervals of about 10 minutes. Each station is likely to consist of a different form of assessment.

Figure 5.1 shows a diagrammatic representation of such a format. A structured interview may be followed by a role-playing station followed by a presentation station. At each station, you will be evaluated by at least two assessors, usually consultants in the specialty. There could be anywhere from three to ten stations altogether.

The list below gives examples of different stations you could expect from a selection centre; all have been used or piloted for ST selection:

- Communication skills station: role-playing scenario
- Presentation station
- Group discussion
- Procedure station, e.g. suturing, intravenous cannulation
- Clinical scenario, e.g. resuscitation scenario, examining patient
- Data interpretation, e.g. chest X-ray, blood results
- Telephone consultation

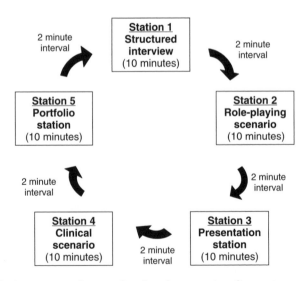

Figure 5.1 A commonly used selection centre format.

- Documentation station: case notes or discharge summary
- Problem solving exercise
- Written exercise, e.g. completing a consultation record

A structured interview is likely in at least one station, but it is unlikely that you will encounter all of the above assessments at any single selection centre. I will elaborate on how to prepare for these different assessment types later in this chapter.

Three golden rules

- Sell yourself
- Maximize your interview score
- Be prepared

Sell yourself

You may be the best doctor in the world, but unless you can demonstrate this to the assessors you won't get the job. Many doctors feel embarrassed about promoting themselves, but interview is a competition. In the more competitive specialties, deaneries aim to interview four candidates for each post available, so you must use every opportunity to sell yourself and make yourself stand out from the crowd.

Selling yourself is not the same as lying—talk about yourself, show your strengths, but **never lie.**

Maximize your interview score

Your performance at interview (or selection centre) will be scored using a marking scheme. This score (in combination with the short-listing score) will determine whether you are offered a job. Be aware of what the marking scheme is going to cover and how you will be assessed to maximize your score. Here are a few suggestions:

- Read the interview marking schemes of those specialties that reveal them. The person specifications for most specialties overlap significantly. Use Google to search for 'interview marking scheme' or 'interview evaluation form'. Use the advanced search function to limit your searches to the domains nhs.uk or ac.uk.
- Use the marking schemes in this book.
- Work out your own interview marking scheme.

In keeping with national regulations, the marking scheme must relate to the person specifications. Table 5.1 shows part of an interview marking scheme that I have derived from person specifications and various published interview marking schemes.[1,2]

Table 5.1 Interview marking scheme: what have you done to find out about the specialty?

Commitment to specialty	Positive indicators	Negative indicators
What have you done to find out about the specialty? **Additional probes** What did you learn from your experience? What are the downsides of this specialty? Have you considered other specialties?	• Substantial effort made to learn about the specialty • Aware of the pros and cons of the specialty • Shows significant thought about specialty choice • Undergraduate prize, distinction, or merit in the specialty • Gives coherent and logical answer	• Little effort made to learn about specialty • Poor insight into pros and cons of the specialty • No significant thought about specialty choice • No achievement related to the specialty • Incoherent or illogical answer
Notes to justify rating	Rating (assessor to allocate rating) 1. Poor 2. Cause for concern 3. Satisfactory 4. Good or excellent	

The more positive indicators that an applicant displays, the higher his or her interview score. Every sample question in **CHAPTER 6** is accompanied by a list of positive indicators. This will give you a flavour of what interviewers are after.

Table 5.2 shows an alternative interview marking scheme (global rating). It should look familiar to you because it is similar to the structured reference forms for referees which are available online from deanery websites.

Be prepared: interviews are like exams

For career progression, succeeding at interviews (or selection centres) is just as important as passing professional exams. Most doctors would start revising for an exam months in advance. You wouldn't expect to pass if you started cramming a fortnight beforehand! Yet, many doctors prepare for interview only when they have been short-listed.

Table 5.2 An alternative interview marking scheme (global rating)

Leadership and teamwork

0	1	2	3	4
No evidence	Does not show any leadership qualities. Is a passive participant and does not engage with team members. Rigid and does not consider the views of team members	Show a little leadership potential. Little initiative shown, with mostly passive participation. Engages with other team members only when required. Limited flexibility and consideration of other team members' views	Show some leadership potential. There is some initiative and active engagement with other team members. Demonstrates some flexibility and considers the views of other team members	Displays strong leadership qualities. Takes initiative and is an active participant. Actively engages with team members. Flexible and considers other members' views

The ideal time to start preparing for interview is a few months beforehand. Create your own preparation schedule and follow it. Use the sample schedule below and in Table 5.3 as a guide. It is important you commit it to paper and give yourself specific and realistic goals.

3–4 MONTHS BEFORE INTERVIEW

- Find out about the interview format (**SEE PAGE 60**) from previous years.
- Research the training programmes in the appropriate deaneries (**SEE PAGE 60**).
- Organize your portfolio (**CHAPTER 3**).
- Form an interview practice group (**SEE PAGE 64**).
- Book an interview preparation course (**SEE PAGE 65**).
- Research issues specific to the specialty (**SEE PAGE 61**).
- Read the latest research and clinical topics in the specialty (**SEE PAGE 61**).

Table 5.3 Sample interview preparation schedule

Weeks before interview	Tasks
13	• Research interview format: e-mail or phone deanery • Organize portfolio; buy stationery and gather competencies, assessments, certificates, etc • Book an interview course
12	• Research interview format: contact current post-holder • Organize portfolio: create contents page, arrange into sections • Organize interview practice group: contact interested colleagues
11	• Research deaneries and training programmes
10	**Application process opens** • Application form • Approach referees
9	• Application form • Get feedback on application form from seniors before submission
8	**Application deadline** • Application form: submission
7	• Interview practice group: first session • Research topical issues (specific to specialty) • Organize portfolio
6	**Annual leave: week off**
5	• Arrange mock interview with consultant • Self-practice: clinical governance, research, teaching • Research topical issues (specific to specialty)
4	• Interview practice group: second practice session • Revise resuscitation manuals (i.e. ALS) and common emergencies • Attend interview course
3	• Interview practice group: third session • Self-practice: commitment to specialty
2	• Arrange practicalities for interview: transport, accommodation, dry-cleaning • Mock interview with consultant/colleague
1	• Self-practice: revise all interview areas • Review portfolio and CV
0	**Interview week** • Final interview preparations

- Arrange a mock interview with consultants **(SEE PAGE 64)**.
- Interview practice group: organize a few sessions.
- Practice answering questions in different areas of the person specifications (read **CHAPTER 6**).
- Review your CV and application form **(SEE PAGE 61)**.
- Revise resuscitation manuals and clinical manuals.
- Prepare for selection centre stations (if relevant).

LESS THAN 1 MONTH BEFORE INTERVIEW

- Make practical arrangements, i.e. travel, accommodation **(SEE PAGE 66)**.
- Final interview question practice.
- Review your CV and portfolio for a final time.

Emergency preparation schedule

This section is for those that have left things to the last minute. If you have only a few days before your interview, don't panic. Leaving things this late isn't ideal but there is still enough time to improve your interview performance. Follow the steps in the emergency preparation schedule below:

- Research the selection process **(PAGE 60)**. You are on a tight schedule and your preparation has to be focused.
- Organize your portfolio. Expect a portfolio station even if you have not been told. For a top portfolio, read **PAGES 22 AND 86**.
- Get the essential paperwork in order. If the documentation you bring to interview is inadequate, you may be refused an interview **(PAGE 66)**.
- If you are attending a selection centre read **CHAPTERS 5 AND 6**. They contain advice on interview and other assessment methods.
- On **PAGES 60 TO 82** of this chapter I give advice on preparing for structured interviews. In **CHAPTER 6** there are sample questions and answers to follow.
- There is specialty-specific advice in **CHAPTER 7**: read the section relevant to your specialty.
- Practice with mock interviews (important!). Read the section 'Practice makes perfect' **(PAGE 64)**.
- Review your application form and portfolio; the interview questions will probably be focused on these.

Prepare strategically: don't just work hard, work smart

Your time is limited and must be used wisely. Your preparation has to be focused and strategic.

Research the interview process

The upcoming interviews are probably going to be similar to those of previous years—redesigning a new interview format is time-consuming and labour-intensive. If you know about the likely interview format and past questions you will have a head start. Your best bet is to ask the current specialty trainees (or anyone else who has been through interviews recently).

Offer to buy them lunch and 'pump' them for information on the format. Approach them face-to-face if you can. Provided you are polite and catch them at a good time, many specialty trainees will be happy to oblige.

You should ask the following sort of questions:

- What was the interview format?
- How many different stations were there and what was covered at each station?
- What assessment methods were used, e.g. role-playing, presentations, practical skills assessment?
- If there was a portfolio station, which part was scrutinized?
- What were the hardest interview questions?

Anticipate interview questions: using the person specifications

Don't try to predict the exact interview questions; it isn't possible. However, it is easy to anticipate which areas the interview questions are likely to evaluate. Your clue is in the person specifications.

Every interview question will evaluate a particular section of the person specifications and every interviewer will be allocated a specific section (or sections) to evaluate. Below, I've listed the main sections of the person specifications from the MMC website.[3] Most of these specifications below are relevant to all specialties.

- Clinical expertise and technical knowledge
- Research skills
- Teaching
- Vigilance and situational awareness
- Coping with pressure
- Managing others and team involvement

- Problem solving and decision making
- Empathy and sensitivity
- Communication skills
- Leadership and team involvement
- Organization and planning
- Professional integrity and respect for others
- Commitment to specialty

For each section above, practice answering several possible questions. With a little adaptation you can use the same answer for different questions. Be systematic and aim to cover all of them. In **CHAPTER 6**, I shall go through each specification with sample questions and answers.

Perform well across the board

You should aim to be equally well prepared for all sections in the person specifications. If a candidate were to perform particularly badly in one section this could make them unappointable even if they excelled elsewhere.[3,4] It is easier to score slightly above average across the board than to attain a perfect score at multiple stations. The highest-scoring candidates are likely to perform well across most areas.

Review your portfolio and CV

Review your portfolio and CV before your interview; you are likely to be quizzed on them at some point and it may have been a while since you looked at them. Going through your portfolio and CV will also give you new inspiration for interview responses.

Know your specialty

Topical questions are very common, and are often on a 'hot topic' or an area of controversy within the specialty. Questions could pertain to newly published guidelines or an exciting area of research. Alternatively, they could be about a regulation such as the '2 week rule' or the European Working Time Directive.

You will only be able to give coherent answers if you have enough background knowledge. Ask consultants and trainees in the specialty what the current 'hot topics' are. Read the relevant royal college's website and newsletters. There should be a 'letters' or 'forum' section. If there is much interest in a topic, it is likely to surface at interview. Do some background reading on these issues and consider different viewpoints. If you have an opinion on a controversial issue make sure you are able to justify it.

You might also be asked to discuss a recent publication or topic of interest in the specialty. Choose three topics that interest you. It could be a novel treatment, new findings on a condition, or the latest clinical guidelines. Make sure your topics are not too broad and read a few different sources for each. I find review papers particularly useful. Reviews can be found on PubMed (www.pubmed.gov) or UpToDate (www.uptodate.com). Your hospital library should also have a collection of journals to access.

Answering well

> ## What makes an excellent interview answer?
>
> Excellent answer = positive indicators
> +
> Personalized
> +
> appropriate tone of voice and facial expression

What are interviewers looking for?

Interviewers will have a marking score sheet. A list of positive indicators usually accompanies each question on the score sheet. The more positive indicators that a candidate demonstrates, the higher their score is likely to be. To guide you, in **CHAPTER 6** I have provided a list of positive indicators for each example question in that chapter. You can derive your own list of positive indicators using the person specifications for your specialty.

Keep your answers personal

You have to 'sell' yourself and you can't do this effectively if you use words like 'we' or 'us'. If your answers consist of generic statements they won't work either. Talk about **YOU and YOUR experiences.** In your answers, make sure you are the centre of attention so you can promote your positive qualities. (See the section on 'Teaching' in **CHAPTER 6 (PAGE 97)** for an example.)

Non-verbal cues: vocal tone and body language

Professional actors do not recite their script in a monotone—their facial expressions and tone of voice also convey the meaning of their words. Likewise, no matter how brilliant your words are at interview, they will fail to be believable if you don't deliver them with the right tone of voice and body language.

The best way to achieve a convincing delivery is to ensure your answers are genuine and come straight from your heart. I know this advice is a bit soppy, but it really is the best way. Professional actors require years of training; what chance have you got? An experienced interviewer can tell if you are bluffing straight away. Of course, if one of your reasons for choosing the specialty was because of the lucrative private practice, you might be better off not mentioning this. Speak the truth, but use your discretion.

Practise answering questions in front of a mirror. Alternatively, use a camera with video function or a web cam. Concentrate on your tone of voice and facial expressions; scrutinize them. Tweak the way you deliver your answer until it appears believable to you.

Here are a few more pointers:

- Look alert and interested when the interviewer is speaking. Deliver your answers with enthusiasm and a little pressure in your speech. Your tone of voice and facial expression should be saying 'I really want this job!'.
- Maintain eye contact with the interviewer asking the question. When responding, maintain this eye contact, but engage other members of the interview panel; they are scoring you too.
- Sit up straight in your chair and lean forward slightly when listening. Do not slouch back into your seat or appear too laid-back.
- Fidgeting during your interview will distract interviewers and may even annoy them. Keep your hands on your lap and don't tap your feet.

Smile and be friendly

The interviewers are choosing their future colleagues. They want trainees with whom they can get along on a daily basis. You will need to come across as someone who's likeable and agreeable professionally. Your likeability is not scored directly, but the interviewers are only human, and scoring has a subjective element.

During your interview, smile, be friendly, and appear approachable. Don't come across as being argumentative, arrogant, or 'high-maintenance'.

Be concise

Many interviewers (myself included) tend to have a drift of attention after a couple of minutes. When this happens, the interviewer will have a glazed-over, expressionless face; he or she has momentarily day-dreamed. Not good! When this happens, your answer is likely to receive an average score at best.

To help prevent this happening I recommend a maximum answer length of 2 minutes. Here are my tips for keeping your answers under the time limit:

- Get straight to the point, answer the question immediately. Avoid going off on a tangent. All of you will have struggled to take histories from patients with verbal diarrhoea. It is hard work and time-consuming. Make it easier for the interviewers to award you points.

- You have a time limit. Make every second count towards promoting yourself.
- Speak at a conversational rate. If you answer in a machine-gun like fashion, the interviewers will struggle to follow you. It is not about cramming in as many words as you can in 2 minutes. It is about making every word count.

Practice makes perfect

You can't learn to be a doctor from a book—you need to meet real patients and put your knowledge into practice. Likewise, if you want to perform well at interview you should practise what you have learnt from this book.

Self-practice

You can practise answering questions on your own. Before you answer, think about the best response. Write down your answer in bullet-point form. When answering, you can elaborate on each point as in a presentation. Do not memorize your answers word-for-word; you will appear mechanical. Verbalize your answers aloud and practice until you are satisfied with your response. Try to speak in a relaxed conversational tone.

The trick is to be prepared but not to appear over-rehearsed. An over-rehearsed performance will make interviewers doubt an applicant. Good interview preparation is like good make-up; if done well it will enhance your appearance, but it must not be too obvious!

Mock interviews

In addition to self-practice, a mock interview is strongly advised. Answering questions in front of another person is not the same as doing it in front of a mirror. Enlist the help of a senior, usually a consultant or registrar in the specialty. Preferably, ask a consultant who has interviewed for specialty training (post-MMC) and is good at giving feedback.

Arrange your mock interview early; I recommend the period after your application form has been submitted and before you receive your invitation to interview. If you wait to be short-listed, the chances are the consultant you had in mind will have been 'booked' by your rivals. After your mock interview ask for feedback and suggestions for improvement.

Interview practice group: the more the merrier

Form your own interview practice group to supplement the mock interview. Enlist three or four like-minded colleagues who are applying to the same grade for a few practice sessions after work. Choose a quiet venue where you can be undisturbed (**not** the ward office or staff room!). Don't forget to bring copious amounts of strong coffee and a few treats!

It doesn't matter if you are applying to different specialties; most interview questions are very similar. The exception is GP applicants who should form their own practice group (see the section on General Practice in **CHAPTER 7**). In your groups, take turns being interviewer and interviewee. Practice one question at a time followed immediately by feedback.

Use the practice questions in **CHAPTER 6**. Each question is followed by a list of positive indicators. The positive indicators are a guide to what interviewers are looking for. Table 5.4 is a feedback form that the 'interviewer' can use for each question. A full-page version can be found in Appendix 3. Feel free to make photocopies of this. Make your feedback constructive and emphasize suggestions for improvement.

Interview courses

There are many courses out there that claim to help you prepare for interviews. Attendance isn't essential, indeed many successful applicants have never been to one. On the other hand, attending a good course may improve your performance and give you an edge. My view is that if you can find a good course and obtain funding for it, then why not?

The majority of courses are run by commercial organizations. You are the customer, so shop around carefully. Not all courses are equal. Lecture-based courses can be

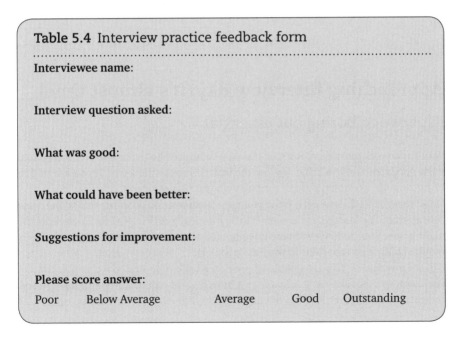

Table 5.4 Interview practice feedback form

Interviewee name:

Interview question asked:

What was good:

What could have been better:

Suggestions for improvement:

Please score answer:

Poor   Below Average   Average   Good   Outstanding

particularly lucrative as they can maximize their revenue and take large numbers of customers. Courses that teach in small groups have to limit their numbers.

You are likely to learn more with interactive (one-to-one or small group teaching) than with didactic teaching. The smaller the teaching group, the more opportunities you will have to practice and ask questions. When choosing a course, keep an eye out for the maximum number of delegates, and if this is not advertised ask the organizers. 'Small-group teaching' can vary anywhere between 5 and 20 delegates.

Below are my suggestions:

- Scrutinize the course itinerary. How much time is allocated for interview practice? How much of it is lecture-based? Do you really need to spend 2 hours on 'hot topics in the NHS?'—this is something you could read about on your own.

- Ask your colleagues for recommendations. How much interview practice did they receive? Did the course help their interview performance on the day?

- Look at the credentials of the course tutors. Have they interviewed for specialty training before?

- Many course websites will display glowing recommendations from previous delegates. These recommendations have been selected by the organizers. The comments of disgruntled customers will not be displayed.

- If an interview course does not advertise the size of its teaching groups, be wary. It might be largely lecture-based or the group sizes could be big. Make sure you check.

- Consider enrolling for a one-to-one interview course. You will have the undivided attention of the tutor and will get the most interview practice.

Approaching interview day: it's almost time!

Paperwork, boring but essential

Your paperwork must be in order or you may be refused an interview. You will be told what documentation to bring. Follow the instructions to the letter. If you are told to bring 'original' documents, don't turn up with just photocopies.

Get this vital task done early on so you can concentrate on other aspects of interview preparation. The last thing you want is to be frantically rummaging for documents the night before your interview. Some documents such as references take time and may require chasing up (consultants are busy people!).

If for any reason you are unable to provide all the requested documents, contact the deanery beforehand. It helps if you have a good explanation and have proof. Suggest an alternative form of documentation. For example, if your passport was stolen, provide a copy of the police report. As an alternative, bring along your driving licence as a form of photo ID or your birth certificate as proof of citizenship.

Looking the part

Even before you sit down, the interviewers will have created their own impressions of you based on your appearance. Creating a good first impression sets the tone for the rest of the interview. Interview scoring has a subjective element as the interviewers are only human. You are likely to score better if you look tidy and professional.

As soon as you enter the room, you want to look believable as a future colleague. For men this means wearing a well-pressed suit, tie, ironed shirt, and polished shoes. Stick to dark or neutral colours at all times. When you leave the room you want the interviewers to talk about your interview performance, not your garish tie. Have a fresh shave and keep your hair tidy.

Women should dress conservatively, avoiding plunging necklines or short skirts. Again, you don't want to distract from your interview performance. It is an urban myth that skirts are preferred; trousers are perfectly acceptable. Remember to keep long hair tied up and avoid excessive make-up. You are auditioning for the role of doctor, not movie star.

Getting there

Work out how you are going to get to the interview venue and estimate the timing of the journey. Leave plenty of extra time for potential delays like congestion and delayed trains. Aim to arrive an hour earlier than your actual interview time.

If your interview is first thing in the morning and is far away, staying overnight at a nearby hotel will minimize the rush-hour stress and ensure you arrive fresh. Being alert on the day may make all the difference between a job offer and a rejection letter.

Know **exactly** where to report to and research how to get there once you arrive. Many interviews are held at very large venues like stadiums with multiple entrances. Bring along a map of the local area and a site map of the venue if you can.

Pack your bags

Create a checklist of all the essential items you need to bring to interview. Pack everything you need before interview day, going through your checklist. Do this one final time, just before you leave. It would be a real shame if you missed your chance because of a forgotten certificate or letter.

On the big day

It is normal to be nervous on interview day; after all, you've waited all year for this. But always keep calm; you need to be sharp and on the ball—if you are a bag of nerves, the adrenaline (or epinephrine!) will mess with your mind.

The best way keep calm is to be well prepared and practiced. You could flip through your portfolio while you wait. Alternatively, concentrate on your breathing and take slow, deep breaths. If talking to other applicants makes you nervous, then sit somewhere else on your own. Don't feel obliged to speak to them.

Remember, you have been through worse than this before. Unlike medical school finals, you won't be jobless if you do badly; there are many non-training jobs you can apply for. Your career won't come to an end; at worst, you will have to reapply next year.

After the interview

Immediately after your interview make a note of all the questions and assessments. If you struggled anywhere, record that too. Write down what you could have done differently or how you could have prepared better. Spend about 15–20 minutes doing this.

It may not seem important now, but these notes will be your insurance policy should you (touch wood!) not get a job. You can use these notes to learn and improve for the next round of interviews. Do not rely on memory; you will forget details, especially after many months. With each interview you attend, you can get better and better.

Check your e-mail daily after your interview. Past candidates have been given just 48 hours to accept or reject an offer. It would be a shame to miss a job because you failed to accept the offer.

Practical skills assessment

This is used by surgical specialties such as Neurosurgery, Urology, Trauma and Orthopaedics, and Cardio-Thoracics.[1] In most cases, suturing or knot-tying is one of the given tasks. The best way to prepare is to practise these skills repeatedly until you can do them automatically. Borrow instruments and suture (with permission) to practise on an orange peel. Get a senior to teach you the correct technique and observe you.

OSATS, or Objective Structured Assessment of Technical Skills, often is used to asses applicants because it is an established measure of technical skill.[1] The OSATS marking scheme consists of the following:[4]

- **Respect for tissue.** Handle tissues carefully, avoid unnecessary force and minimize damage. Use the correct instruments when handling tissue.
- **Time and motion.** Move efficiently, avoid unnecessary moves (economy of motion).
- **Instrument handling.** Keep your motions fluid. Avoid appearing hesitant.
- **Knowledge of instruments.** Be familiar with instruments and their names. Use instruments appropriately.

- **Flow of operation.** Move smoothly from one part of the procedure to the next. Avoid hesitant stops.
- **Knowledge of specific procedure.** Be fluent and familiar with the procedure.

The ability to perform the procedure accounts for only part of the assessment. Don't neglect the following areas:

- Obtain consent and explain the procedure
- Give effective analgesia (local anaesthetic)
- Use aseptic technique and wash hands
- Dispose of sharps/instruments
- Complete documentation
- Give instructions to patient post-procedure

OSCE: history or examination

Clinical scenarios tend to contain more than one facet to a problem. In addition to the clinical aspect, there are psycho-social and ethical dilemmas. The better candidates will pick up on this and address them.

For example, a young man presents looking unkempt with 2 months of weight loss, night sweats, and cough. TB is a possibility. Consider asking about housing (homeless?), illicit drug use, alcohol, and close contacts.

The best candidates also think like consultants. In addition to the acute management they consider the longer-term management, patient education, and follow-up arrangements. An example is a patient with an exacerbation of asthma. Don't just stop at your management of the acute phase, but consider the longer-term picture like education on inhaler technique, smoking cessation, reviewing steroid inhaler dose, respiratory nurse follow-up etc.

Here are a few more pointers:

- Follow the instructions carefully. Are you asked to focus on a particular part of the history?
- There are usually clues in the instructions. For example, if asked to take a history from a man found sleeping rough and looking dishevelled, the social, alcohol, and drug history is important.
- Introduce yourself and obtain consent. Always be friendly and polite.
- When examining, expose and position the patient correctly.
- At the end, offer to answer any questions the patient may have. Remember to thank the patient when you are finished.
- Without prompting, summarize your findings concisely—positive findings and important negative findings together with your management plan.

- Follow up with the most likely diagnoses and your immediate management plan in a confident manner.
- Don't be fazed if your examiner has a cool or neutral expression. This isn't finals; they aren't there to cheer you on.

Presentation station

You might only be told about this on interview day, hence the importance of researching the selection process. If applicants from previous years had a presentation, then you ought to prepare in advance.

Even if there was no presentation station in the past, always have a couple of specialty topics ready before your interview. Have at least one clinical condition and one research area. Choose a clinical condition that isn't too broad and can realistically be covered in a couple of days. For example, if attending Cardiology interviews, broad topics like 'heart failure' or 'ischaemic heart disease' are too ambitious. Choose focused topics such as dilated cardiomyopathy or the management of ST elevation MI.

The most time-efficient way to prepare is to read review papers on the topic. eMedicine (emedicine.medscape.com) contains thousands of reviews and is free after registration. Google Scholar (scholar.google.co.uk) also has free review articles.

Applicants are scored on the following criteria:

1. **Organization of presentation.** Your overheads should be easy to read. Don't cram excessive words onto each slide. Use 'bullet points', but no more than four per slide. Talk around each bullet point and do not read out your slides.
2. **Communication skills.** You will be judged on your ability to be understood and communicate your ideas effectively. Your speech should be clear, projected, and not too fast. Engage your audience by maintaining eye contact and using hand gestures.
3. **Time management.** You will be penalized if your presentation overshoots or is far too short. If you were allocated 10 minutes, aim for a presentation of 8–9 minutes. Practise with a stopwatch, and during your presentation keep an eye on the time. If your watch has a 'countdown' function, program it to ring 2 minutes before the end.
4. **Content.** Choose a topic that is relevant to the specialty or in line with instructions. You must have a good knowledge and depth of understanding of the topic.
5. **Questioning.** Sometimes time is allocated for questioning after the interview. You will be marked on your ability to communicate with the interviewers and how well you know the topic you have presented.

Clinical scenario—resuscitation

If you are applying for an acute specialty, be prepared for a resuscitation scenario. Revise resuscitation manuals and common emergencies in your specialty.

During the scenario, keep calm; you need to think logically. Systematically go through the protocol you were taught. You have managed real emergencies before; imagine yourself at work. Below are key points to remember:

- Summon help immediately, i.e. alarm cord, fast bleep, arrest call.
- Remember the basics; airway, breathing, circulation, **focused** history, and examination.
- Re-assess the patient, particularly if there is a change in condition.
- Involve other specialties if appropriate, e.g. anaesthetist, physician, paediatrician.
- Contact other team members and seniors if needed.

If the 'patient' deteriorates or something goes wrong don't be fazed; this might well be part of the scenario and it doesn't necessarily reflect on your performance. After the station, try not to think too hard about it and focus on the next station. If you found the scenario challenging, it is likely that other applicant will too. **CHAPTER 7** will cover common clinical scenarios for each specialty.

Role-playing scenario

Role-playing scenarios are used for testing an applicant's communication skills. You will be given a scenario based on real-life situations; it usually is relevant to the specialty. Scenarios are usually:

- breaking bad news
- explaining a diagnosis or results
- dealing with complaints or disgruntled relatives
- explaining procedures or treatment options
- patient education

You will gain the most if you practise with colleagues or in your interview practice groups. Take turns at being actor and doctor. Use the practice scenarios provided below. **CHAPTER 7** contains additional scenarios for each specialty; work through those too.

Table 5.5 shows a marking scheme proforma derived from interview evaluation forms and person specifications.[1,2] Each scenario is accompanied by a list of 'positive indicators'. Use it to help mark your performance. Here are a few pointers:

- Read the instructions carefully. Identify your main task and try to avoid being side-tracked during the scenario.

Table 5.5 Role-play marking scheme

Role-play scenario

Introduction and closure	**3 Points**

- Introduces self and role
- Summarizes
- Closes scenario appropriately

Listening	**3 Points**

- Actively listens
- Allows time for questions
- Identifies and explores concerns and issues

Verbal	**3 Points**

- Uses everyday language
- Minimizes use of jargon, explains any used
- Clear and easily understood

Non-verbal	**3 Points**

- Appropriate eye contact, tone of voice, and body language
- Not-condescending or confrontational
- Adapts to patient's response and emotions

Positive indicators (accompanies each scenario)	**5 Points**
Total score	**/18 Points**

Suggestions for improvement

- At the start always introduce yourself and explain your presence to the patient. Also confirm the patient's name.
- Minimize the use of jargon and explain any technical terms you use in every-day language.
- Expect the unexpected. If the patient goes into a rage or sobs hysterically, this is probably part of the script and not a reflection of your performance. Do what you **ought** to do in real life. Adapt to the situation. If you were instructed to take a history but the patient is bawling, you need to change your approach. Console the patient and resume only when he or she is settled.

- Towards the end of the scenario, offer to answer any questions the patient has. Marking schemes also score closure, so a brief summary is important.
- If appropriate, arrange further follow-up in clinic or with a nurse specialist.
- If explaining a diagnosis or breaking bad news, give further sources of information such as booklets, websites, or charitable organizations.

Scenario 1

CANDIDATE INSTRUCTIONS

You are the orthopaedic ST1 and Mr Bearn, a 79-year-old man, was admitted for an elective hip replacement. The procedure itself was uncomplicated, but a few days later Mr Bearn developed diarrhoea. A stool specimen has confirmed *Clostridium difficile* toxin. Mr Bearn has been on metronidazole for 2 days as advised by the microbiologist. He is slightly delirious and the diarrhoea is still present.

Mr Bearn's daughter has just arrived from Australia. She is on the ward and demands to speak to the doctor. Your task is to speak to the daughter and update her on her father's condition. You are expected to respond appropriately to any questions or concerns raised.

You have a total of 10 minutes, including 2 minutes of reading time.

SUGGESTED RESPONSE

DR CHARNLEY: Hello, are you Ms Bearn? Good morning. My name is Dr Charnley. I am a specialty trainee in Orthopaedics and am one of the doctors looking after your father. How can I help?

[Check you have the right person. Always greet and introduce yourself. Explain why you are there.]

MS BEARN: Finally! I have been waiting for over 45 minutes to speak to a doctor. What is going on with my father? He looks dreadful!

[Ms Bearn is clearly irate; this is part of the script. You will be judged on how you deal with this emotion. Defuse the anger by apologizing early on. Stay calm and lower the tone of your voice.]

DR CHARNLEY: I do apologize for keeping you waiting. It has been busy but I came to see you as soon as I could…[Ms Bearn abruptly interrupts]

MS BEARN: What has happened to my father? What have you done to him? He was perfectly well before he came to hospital.

[Do not get provoked by Ms Bearn's interruption. Check what the patient or relative knows. I recommend this in most role-playing scenarios. They may have been misinformed and this may reveal the root of their anxiety.]

DR CHARNLEY: What have you been told so far about your father?

MS BEARN: I know that my father came into hospital a healthy man for a planned hip replacement. Now he has caught diarrhoea from this hospital.

DR CHARNLEY: Your father was admitted to hospital 5 days ago for a planned hip replacement. The procedure itself went according to plan and there were no complications on the day. Unfortunately, he developed diarrhoea a few days after the procedure. We have tested his stool and it has come back positive for a bacterium called Clostridium difficile or C. difficile for short. Have you heard of C. difficile before?

[If you use any jargon always offer to explain it, but be careful not to be condescending.]

MS BEARN: Yes I have! It has been in the news a lot recently. I know that you get it from filthy hospitals like this one. That is why my father has caught C. difficile. This is your fault!

[An outburst of anger followed by an accusation. Do not get defensive or confrontational as this is counterproductive. Always stay calm and lower the tone of your voice. Ms Bearn is upset. Try to empathize with her and show some sympathy. Apologizing does not necessarily mean admitting guilt.]

DR CHARNLEY: I know you are angry and I probably would feel the same way if in your situation. I am truly sorry about your father's illness. Would you want a little time to yourself before we continue talking?

[If clearly disturbed, offer Ms Bearn time to compose herself]

MS BEARN: No, I am fine. Carry on.

DR CHARNLEY: Please, let me explain a little more about your father's illness. C. difficile is a bacterium that occurs naturally in the human gut. It is found in about 1 in 20 people in the community. In healthy people it doesn't usually cause problems. This is because other bacteria in the gut keep it under control. In patients who have received antibiotics, the usual bacteria living in the gut are affected. In some patients, particularly the elderly, C. difficile in the gut could multiply and cause diarrhoea.

Do you have any questions about what I have explained so far? Please feel free to ask if anything is unclear.

MS BEARN: I understand everything. Please continue.

[Use everyday language to explain jargon and technical concepts. Intermittently, check that the daughter understands.]

DR CHARNLEY: In your father's case, he received a short course of antibiotics as a routine part of his hip replacement. Research has shown that administering antibiotics during a hip replacement reduces the risk of a joint infection. From our experience, a short course of antibiotics does not lead to problems in the vast majority of patients. Unfortunately in your father's situation, this has not been the case.

[Later in the scenario, check if Ms Bearn has further concerns. If there are any, the actor usually tries to help by hinting. Explore what these concerns could be. If there is time, try to summarize the meeting in a few lines. Offer Ms Bearn a means of contacting you for future meetings.]

POSITIVE INDICATORS

- Deals with anger appropriately: apologizes, sympathizes
- Does not get angry, defensive, or confrontational
- Demonstrates understanding and empathy
- Does not blame colleagues
- Takes action on concerns

Scenario 2

CANDIDATE INSTRUCTIONS

Last week, 45-year-old Mrs Gray noticed a lump in her left breast. She was sent for a mammogram which has just been reported. You are the doctor seeing her in clinic. Please explain the results of the mammogram and recommended investigations to her. You are to respond to her concerns. Do **not** take a history.

Mammogram report: suspicious abnormality of undetermined significance in the left breast. Recommend further investigation.

PATIENT INSTRUCTIONS

You recently felt a lump in your left breast, but didn't make much of it. You are attending clinic, expecting the 'all clear' from your doctor.

Five years ago, your mother died from breast cancer at the age of 70, despite a disfiguring mastectomy. At the back of your mind, you are worried that you could have inherited this from her. You are terrified of needles and procedures because of the pain they can cause. Do not express any of your concerns to the doctor unless he or she asks.

POSITIVE INDICATORS

- Breaks the news gently and sensitively
- Displays empathy and concern
- Explains needle biopsy in everyday language

- Identifies and explores fear of inherited cancer
- Identifies and explores fear of needles

Scenario 3

Candidate instructions

Mr Cushing is an 18-year-old man who presented with a severe headache that started suddenly at the back of his head. He thought his vision briefly became blurred, but this has now resolved. He has had a full neurological examination which was unremarkable. A CT brain scan was reported as normal by the radiologist. Your consultant has asked you to perform a lumbar puncture on Mr Cushing to rule out a subarachnoid haemorrhage.

Your task is to explain the lumbar puncture to him and obtain his consent. Respond to his concerns as appropriate.

Instructions to actor playing Mr Cushing

You have had a splitting headache for 2 days now. Despite the painkillers, you are still in agony and also feel very nauseated. You don't know what the fuss is about and why you have to be in hospital. As far as you are concerned this headache is just a migraine. You overheard the nurse saying that the lumbar puncture was being done because the doctor 'needed practice'. You don't want to be a guinea pig for the lumbar puncture and have no idea what it involves. You will only agree to the test if the doctor can give you a good reason for it. Otherwise, you are going to discharge yourself today.

Positive indicators

- Explains reasons for lumbar puncture
- Describes seriousness of subarachnoid haemorrhage
- Explains procedure to patient in everyday language
- Offers additional analgesia and anti-emetics to relieve symptoms
- Explores reasons for patient refusal
- Discusses or offers alternative investigation, e.g. MRI brain
- 'Procedure practice' allegation: offers to investigate but does not blame staff

Scenario 4

Candidate instructions

Mrs Glen is an 88-year-old woman with vascular dementia. She lives at home with her daughter who is her main carer. Mrs Glen is fully dependent on her daughter for all personal needs. She is chair- or bed-bound and is not mobile. She has been admitted with septicaemia secondary to a urinary tract infection. Despite antibiotics and aggressive fluid resuscitation she remains profoundly hypotensive and is very ill. You are to speak to her daughter and explain the poor prognosis. Your consultant also wants you to discuss a Do Not Resuscitate Order.

ACTOR INSTRUCTIONS

You are deeply attached to your mother and feel that the doctors are giving up on her because of her age. It makes you angry. You want her to be moved to the intensive care unit and be resuscitated if her heart stops as this will save her life. It usually works on TV!

POSITIVE INDICATORS

- Explain in everyday language, minimal jargon
- Be sympathetic and show empathy
- Explain poor outcome and futility of CPR
- Explores daughter's concerns and beliefs
- Aware that doctor has the final say if the patient is incapacitated

CHAPTER 7 has more specialty-relevant scenarios you can practice.

Group discussion

Public Health use this form of assessment. Until recently, General Practice used this too. In groups of four to six, applicants have about 20 minutes to hold a discussion which will be observed by assessors. Beforehand, applicants are given instructions and a list of issues to cover. Examples include: dealing with an underperforming colleague, responding to a list of complaints from patients, or implementing new policies or deciding how to allocate funds.

During the task, assessors will record your actions against a checklist. This checklist is used to allocate you a score for each attribute.[6] Below is a checklist to give you an idea of what assessors look for and tips on how to improve your performance. This checklist is based on different sources involved in GP training or selection.[5,7]

The best way to prepare is to practise a few different scenarios with a group of colleagues. An alternative is to join a reputable course.

Empathy and sensitivity

- Direct the conversation when required (but do not dominate). Be careful not to be too quiet or too loud.
- Always be polite, friendly, and non-confrontational.
- Treat others as individuals. Call them by name, introduce yourself, and listen to them.
- Focuses on positive rather than negative. Be encouraging.

Communication skills

- Actively listen to others.
- Involve others in discussion, i.e. encourage quieter participants 'what do you think?'.
- Read and use body language, i.e. good eye contact, nod when listening.
- Be welcoming and positive to ideas proposed by others.
- Can form working relationships.
- Respect views of others even if you disagree: 'That's an interesting thought'.
- Speak clearly and audibly to be heard by assessors.

Problem solving

- Identify key points in a problem and prioritize information.
- Be open to others' suggestions. Listen and voice your support if you agree.
- Formulate a workable plan of action.
- Think beyond the obvious. For example, a colleague who is repeatedly late for work could just be lazy, but there may be an underlying personal problem that needs exploring.
- Lateral thinking. Suggest alternative solutions to a problem.

Personal integrity

- Be able to deal with different personality types.
- Enthusiastic and positive when dealing with problems.
- Shows respect for others.
- Appreciates contribution of others.
- Shows respect for the marginalized in society, e.g. drug addicts, homeless.

Prioritization exercise (written)

This is a paper-based exercise which is used by General Practice. Applicants are given a scenario with several incidents taking place simultaneously. You have 20 minutes to rank these incidents in order of priority, explaining your choices. This is followed by a few reflective questions.

To perform well you must provide a comprehensive explanation for how you prioritized. Providing a ranking alone is not enough. Like solving a maths problem, you must show how you derived your answer. Take the time to give a thorough explanation.

- Be able to prioritize issues according to the urgency and importance of tasks. Categorize all your scenarios as follows: emergency (immediate risk to life), urgent (possible risk to life), or routine (unlikely risk to life).
- Remember to ask for help. If your registrar is busy consider others such as your consultant, other specialties, the site manager, your juniors, nurses, or allied health professionals.
- Generate solutions and suggest new ideas to manage dilemmas.
- Make it clear what the key concern is with each incident, i.e. patient at immediate risk or important issue but can be dealt with routinely.
- You are judged on the clarity of your verbal communication. Write legibly and express yourself clearly.
- The reflective questions at the end of the exercise are part of your assessment. You need to show that you are reflective by learning from the scenario and acknowledging your limitations.

Below is a mock scenario with sample answer. There is no 'correct' ranking. What is important is justifying your actions and communicating this clearly.

Scenario

You are the Accident and Emergency F2 on night duty. Your registrar is currently busy with a patient in minors.

A. The charge nurse demands you fill in your discharge summaries from the day before. They have to be sent out by post to the GPs.

B. A nurse passes you a message. It is your partner. It is important that you call back.

C. Paramedics bring in a 9-year-old asthmatic with breathlessness. He is wheezy but talking in full sentences and asking for his mother.

D. An elderly patient with pneumonia has been accepted by the medical team. She was talking 30 minutes ago, but is now unresponsive.

E. A drug addict with a serious paracetamol overdose is threatening to self-discharge within 15 minutes.

Please rank your choices in order with your explanations.

Sample answer

D Likely life-threatening. May have gone into cardio-respiratory arrest. Must repeat primary survey and resuscitate. [Purposely vague with minimal information. Be able to recognize the potential for a life-threatening event.] Fast bleep or cardiac arrest call to medics. Summon your registrar from minors to help with the other cases. [Shows your ability to call for help.]

E Potentially life-threatening overdose. Patient's life at risk if he discharges and this needs to be seen to quickly. Ask for help from registrar or charge nurse to speak to him. [Treat all fairly, including the marginalized members of society.]

C Not life-threatening exacerbation as patient is talking. But should be seen soon as he could deteriorate quickly. Needs observing and treatment with nebulizers. Paediatricians or nurse practitioner could be called to assist. [Think of solutions to managing the situation.]

B You partner rarely calls you at work. It must be important. You take the call once none of your patients are at risk. Also, thinking about it may impinge on your ability to concentrate. [Assessors are looking for applicants who can balance their work/personal commitments. Ignoring your partner is not recommended.]

A Good note-keeping and correspondence are important for patient care. But this is the least urgent task and can wait till the end of the shift.

Telephone consultation

Neurosurgery, Plastic, and Trauma and Orthopaedic surgery have used this assessment method.[1] Applicants are given an imaginary scenario and asked to discuss a emergency over the telephone with a consultant. This station could cover different scenarios such as: making a referral, requesting an urgent scan, or talking to a general practitioner.

The person on the phone will be instructed to be rude or unhelpful; this is part of the script. If the advice over the phone is inappropriate, you **must** raise your concern and hold your ground, even if it is from a consultant. Always be firm but polite. Below are a few scenarios you can practice with colleagues.

The scenario will evaluate applicants in a number of ways:

1. Time-management: you will have a fixed time (10–15 minutes) for the entire station including reading the instructions. You have to assimilate the information and formulate a management plan within this time. Whilst reading instructions, make a list of objectives. Applicants who fail to complete the station will be penalized.

2. Communication skills: you will be judged on how clearly and effectively you communicate. There is a lot of information to convey in a limited time frame. Be concise and give **only** relevant and important information.

    Start by identifying yourself and explain why you are calling, 'Hello, my name is Dr Maxwell, surgical ST1 on-call. Could I discuss a patient who I am concerned about?'. Follow-up with a 'headline' sentence, before going into further detail. 'My patient is a 40-year-old man from an RTA with serious intra-abdominal injuries and requires emergency surgery.'

3. Decision-making: can you prioritize the issues and formulate a rational management plan? Remember the basics, resuscitate the patient and ensure they are stable first. Then list the outstanding issues, describing the most urgent ones first.

4. Organizational skills: remember to involve other professionals as appropriate, e.g. radiology, anaesthesia, transfusion. Are there vital practical tasks such as informing theatre?

Question 1

You are the ST3 on-call and it is midnight. A 45-year-old patient has necrotizing fasciitis in her right lower limb. You have 5 minutes to read the notes and formulate a plan. You are then to call your consultant Mr Gruff with your plan. [Note: Do not expect Mr Gruff to be friendly. This is intentional.]

Positive indicators

- Clear communication
- Resuscitation and sensible plan
- Teamwork, i.e. anaesthetist, theatres, juniors
- Is firm with a 'difficult' consultant

Question 2

Speak to the consultant for Neuro-ITU and ask for a bed for one of your patients. The consultant could challenge you on your appropriateness of your referral or that he would like to 'reserve' his remaining ITU bed.

Question 3

Speak to the neurosurgical consultant on-call (a locum) to come in to help you with an operation that you are not competent with. The procedure is urgent but the consultant might try to persuade you to postpone it.

REFERENCES

1 JCST (Joint Committee on Surgical Training) Good Practice Toolkit. Phase 3: Selection Centre Guidance (www.jcst.org).

2 Royal College of Paediatrics and Child Health National (England and Wales). Selection 2009, interview process and scoring system (www.rcpch.ac.uk).

3 Modernising Medical Careers (www.mmc.nhs.uk).

4 Royal College of Radiologists (2010). Specialty Recruitment [clinical radiology] (http://www.rcr.ac.uk/content.aspx?PageID=1643)

5 Reznick R *et al.* (1997). Testing technical skill via an innovative 'bench station' examination. *American Journal of Surgery*, **173**, 226–230.

6 *A candidate's guide to the selection process for GP specialty training in the London/ KSS Joint UoA. March 2007. London Deanery.*

7 *General Practice specialty training programme Stage 3 selection centre guide 2010. East Midland Deanery.*

CHAPTER 6

Interview: practice questions and answers

How to use this chapter

This chapter has practice questions which have frequently cropped up at ST interviews in previous years. It is divided into sections according to the person specifications. Each section has practice interview questions with accompanying responses, explanations, and positive indicators. Many specialties use positive indicators in their interview marking scheme. The more positive indicators you demonstrate, the higher you score for each question.[1, 2, 3]

Before your interview, practise answering the questions, preferably with a partner or in your interview practice groups. The 'interviewer' can use the feedback form (Table 6.1) for each question practised. Use the positive indicators provided as a marking guide. A full-page version can be found in Appendix 4. Feel free to make photocopies of this page for your personal use.

Don't use the responses in this chapter at your interview. As I mentioned in **CHAPTER 5**, your responses must be personal and reflect your experiences for them to be effective. The examples below are illustrative and aren't perfect. With a little thought, I'm sure you can improve on them. Always be honest in your responses and don't be tempted to make things up. Get caught lying and your chances will disappear faster than you can say 'GMC hearing'.

> **Table 6.1** Interview question feedback form
>
> ....
>
> **Interviewee name:**
>
> **Interview question asked:**
>
> **What was good (i.e. positive indicators demonstrated):**
>
> **What needs improvement (i.e. positive indicators *not* demonstrated):**
>
> **Other suggestions for improvement:**
>
> **Please score answer:**
>
> | Poor | Below average | Average | Good | Outstanding |
> |------|---------------|---------|------|-------------|
> | 1 point | 2 points | 3 points | 4 points | 5 points |

Background question

Question 1

Please tell me about your training and portfolio to date.

POOR RESPONSE

[F2 applying to ST1 in Core Medical Training]

> I studied Medicine at Oxford University and after graduation went on to Foundation Training. My Foundation Training has included posts at the John Radcliffe and Milton Keynes Hospital. I've worked in a wide variety of specialties including Medicine, Anaesthetics, Surgery, and Emergency Medicine. During this time, I've managed a wide variety of cases and have passed my Advanced Life Support Course. I am competent at managing acutely ill patients independently. I've applied to the Core Medical Training programme as I wish to pursue my career as a physician.

NOTE

There is usually an opening question of this type at the beginning of an interview. For the interviewer, it is a handy way of getting an overview of the candidate. A common error is to mechanically talk through your CV or chronologically go through your previous posts. Sure, you are answering the question. But you aren't distinguishing yourself.

The response above is very average because it fails to make the applicant stand out. Every F2 will have worked in a variety of specialties and should be capable of managing acutely ill patients by this stage. Many will be trained in ALS.

This is your chance to make a good first impression and set the right tone for the rest of your interview. You want to get the interviewers thinking, 'Wow! I really want this person to work for me!'. How do you achieve this?

1. **Bring out your distinguishing points**. Have you noticed how shops display their most enticing products in their front window? Likewise, you need to display your distinguishing points prominently. Average isn't good enough; if you want the job you have to be above average. Below are some particularly distinguishing points:
   - *Prestigious or medical finals prizes*
   - *First-class degree*
   - *Presentations at regional, national, or international meetings*
   - *Publications in major journals*
   - *Professional exams such as MRCP, MRCS*
   - *Achievements requiring significant effort such as an MD, PhD, publications, LAT posts, specialty-specific skills and courses.*

2. **Structure your answer**. Structure your answer so that it is logical and brings out your distinguishing points early on. It need not be chronological. For example, if you are strong in research and publications, you could start off with your career ambitions followed by a **brief** summary of your training posts. Link you career ambition with your research and publications. Then move on to other aspects of your CV. Make sure you link your answer to the specialty. This is only a suggestion and it is up to you on how to structure it.

GOOD RESPONSE

I graduated from Oxford two years ago with first-class honours and a medical finals prize. During my Foundation Training I applied to sit for the MRCP membership exam at the earliest possible opportunity. I passed part 1 at my first attempt and am currently revising Part 2 which I plan to sit in 3 months' time.

I have enjoyed my experience working in Medicine. Recently I have presented in a grand round and last year completed an audit. I intend to pursue a career in Infectious Disease. I have recently had a 'taster' post in the specialty. I am applying for this CMT rotation as the next step forward in pursuing my goal.

The majority of doctors do not posses a first-class degree or a medical finals prize. Most F2s will not have passed MRCP part 1. Many candidates let themselves down by significantly underselling themselves. Everybody has different strengths to display. Consider what yours are and bring them out in your response. For example, if you have made many specialty-related presentations or publications, mention it.

Portfolio station

The portfolio station can account for a significant chunk of your interview score; up to a third in some cases. Be well-versed on portfolio and work-based assessments—I suggest you visit the JRCPTB and London Deanery websites (www.jrcptb.org.uk and www.faculty.londondeanery.ac.uk). In your response, always relate back to **your** portfolio.

Your portfolio is evidence of your competencies and training; it represents you. Keep it organized and tidy. An organized portfolio can be your ally at interview. If asked, 'How do we know you are good at teaching?' your response could be, 'I have taught many students and the feedback I have received demonstrates that I am an excellent teacher. I have proof of these in my portfolio here. Would you like to have a look?'.

The scoring at portfolio stations is often based on:

1. **Presentation and organization of portfolio.** This reflects on your organizational and record-keeping skills. Advice on organizing your portfolio is given in **CHAPTER 3**.

2. **Quality of the evidence provided.** The more competencies that you can provide evidence for, the better. For example, if you are applying to Anaesthetics (ST3), competencies in Obstetric Anaesthesia, primary FRCA or Intensive Care Medicine would be desirable. Have a completed log book and a range of work-based assessments. If your portfolio is looking rather thin here, get more assessments before interview.

3. **Questions on training and achievements.** Use your knowledge of the interview scoring system (provided in this chapter) to maximize your score. When asked about an audit you participated in, you earn additional points for playing a lead role, designing it, presenting it, proposing changes, and closing the cycle. Be familiar with the contents of your portfolio and CV.

4. **Knowledge of work-based assessments.** The interviewer may ask your opinion on DOPs, CEX, MSF, MBD etc. Interviewers are looking for candidates with a positive outlook who are certain of their contribution to training. Criticizing the system will get you nowhere.

Question 1

Tell me about your portfolio and its role.

RESPONSE

My portfolio serves as an important record of my training. It records the progress I make through my career and documents the competencies I have achieved. This record is in the form of supervisors' reports, work-based assessments, reflections, and personal development plans. It is also a prospective tool and I find it useful in planning my career.

In addition, I find it very useful as a training aid to identify my strengths and weaknesses. The work-based assessments in my portfolio provide me with suggestions for improvement. For example, I had a mini-CEX of my management of a patient with coeliac disease. The feedback was that my communication skills were good and I was able to empathize with the patient. It also suggested that I should improve my theoretical knowledge of the condition. I made it a point of revising about coeliac disease. I always try to follow the suggestions made, so I can continually improve myself.

NOTES

Don't regurgitate the definition of a portfolio. As in the example above, relate your answer to **your** portfolio. Talk about how you have learnt from your portfolio and the benefits you have reaped.

Scoring systems favour candidates who are positive and benefit from their portfolio. All criticism should be limited and constructive. This is not Speaker's Corner, mind your tongue!

POSITIVE INDICATORS

- Good understanding of a portfolio
- Understands the benefits and importance of a portfolio
- Has learnt or changed practice from a portfolio
- Offers constructive criticism
- Positive outlook

Question 2

Which type of work-based assessment do you find the most useful and why?

RESPONSE

I find the Multi-Source Feedback particularly useful as it gives me an overview picture of myself from colleagues from completely different disciplines. I know

MSF has been shown to be a reliable and accurate tool, particularly if there are at least eight assessors.

In a MSF in my Foundation Year 1, my assessors described that I was approachable and professional at all times. However, a few assessors said that at times I could be quiet and should be more assertive. I have taken this on board and enrolled myself on a leadership course for doctors. Since then, I have taken up leadership roles by being the Doctor's Mess president and trainee representative on the specialty training committee. I believe that I've learnt to become more assertive with colleagues whilst still treating them in a courteous way. I look forward to my next MSF to see how I have progressed.

NOTE

Your response should be personal and describe specific examples. Try to choose an example where you have learnt from your assessment and changed your practice as a result of it.

POSITIVE INDICATORS

- Gives cohesive and logical reasoning
- Has learnt or changed practice as a result of assessment
- Insight into own strengths and weaknesses
- Positive outlook

Question 3

Looking at your training to date, what achievements are you most proud of and why?

RESPONSE

I was the organizer of the Medicine Revision Week course for final year medical students from UCL. It was a significant responsibility, as I was responsible for their training only weeks before their final exams. I had to design a timetable from scratch, book venues, prepare handouts and liaise with consultants throughout. During the week, a tutor became unavailable at the last minute, but fortunately I already had a contingency tutorial in place. I received fantastic feedback from the students at the end of the week, and some of their feedback is in my portfolio here.

Being course organizer was hard work, but I demonstrated my ability to organize and plan effectively. As a consultant physician in future, I would have to plan my team's work schedule effectively in order to ensure good patient care. In addition, 1 gained valuable management and leadership experience. As an aspiring physician, I will be required to manage teams of doctors and have a lead role in clinical care. Dealing with last minute absences demonstrates my ability to problem-solve, another essential skill for an acute physician.

NOTE

The key to performing well here is to relate your achievement to your chosen career. Talk about what you have gained and explain how it is an asset for the specialty. It helps if you have an exceptional achievement. But even if your achievement is modest, you can still perform well.

POSITIVE INDICATORS

- Significant or exceptional achievement(s) for stage of training
- Relates achievement to career in specialty
- Understands relevant strengths for specialty
- Communicates clearly and uses examples

Question 4

Tell me about your experiences of reflective practice.

NOTE

You should have examples of reflective practice in your portfolio, even if not stipulated. Be ready to discuss them and the lessons you have drawn. For a refresher on reflective practice, visit www.foundationprogramme.nhs.uk and download the 'Foundation Learning Portfolio'.

POSITIVE INDICATORS

- Gives specific examples of reflective practice
- Written/typed reflective practice in portfolio
- Understands importance and benefits of reflective practice
- Learns from reflective practice

Question 5

What is the purpose of keeping a portfolio?

POSITIVE INDICATORS

- Good understanding of portfolio
- Understands it as a tool for training and a record of progression
- Cites personal examples of use
- Learns and benefits from portfolio
- Offers constructive criticism (if any)
- Positive outlook

Question 6

What are your main weaknesses?

POSITIVE INDICATORS

- Displays good self-awareness
- Understands own limitations
- Give specific examples
- Learns from weaknesses
- Takes steps to improve and work on weaknesses
- Has positive approach to limitations

Clinical scenarios

For many specialties, a clinical scenario is a major part of the interview. Scenarios will be specialty specific and I have provided clinical scenarios (with marking schemes) for each specialty in **CHAPTER 7**. Expect them to be challenging.

My advice for preparing for such scenarios is threefold:

1. **Revise.** Read resuscitation protocols and common emergencies. Also review conditions that are common or important. For example, aspiring paediatricians should revise asthma, croup, and non-accidental injury. For Trauma and Orthopaedics, open fractures, fractured neck of femur, and wrist fractures.

2. **Practice** the clinical scenarios in **CHAPTER 7** preferably with a colleague or in your interview practice groups. Create your own clinical scenarios. Alternatively, ask a senior to go through a few practice scenarios with you. To keep it realistic, insist on interview-like conditions.

3. **Think ahead**. Always consider the long-term management and fol-low-up. There are multiple facets to every clinical scenario, e.g. social, housing, illicit drugs. To illustrate, for an exacerbation of asthma you should consider smoking cessation, inhaler technique, compliance with medication, pets, housing, and follow-up (nurse-led or in outpatients). If you know about guidelines or the evidence base for management, dis-cuss them to impress.

Here are a few more tips to remember:

- Patient safety must come first. Always ensure the patient is stable first. If not, resuscitate (ABC) and escalate care.
- Remain calm and focused. You have probably encountered a similar case in real life.
- Spend a few moments thinking before you blurt out your answer.

- Sometimes there is no 'correct' way to manage the scenario. The interviewers want to see if you have a safe and logical approach to the scenario.
- As in a clinical exam, respond with confidence and clarity in your voice. Waver and your response will be in doubt, even if it is correct.
- Be systematic and logical in your approach. History, examination, and investigations followed by your differential diagnosis.
- Perform basic investigations before more expensive and invasive ones.
- Be holistic. Consider home situation, family support, alcohol, illicit drugs.
- Involve other specialties if appropriate.
- Involve your seniors when appropriate.

Commitment to specialty

Question 1

Why have you chosen this specialty?

POOR RESPONSE

Anaesthetics has always been at the forefront of innovation and utilizing new technology to benefit patients. It is also an acute specialty with patients who can be very ill and can deteriorate rapidly. Important decisions sometimes have to be made quickly. This makes it at times a challenging but exciting specialty.

Anaesthetics is a multidisciplinary specialty with work in many areas such as surgery, obstetrics, ITU, paediatric cardiology, invasive radiology and chronic pain. This gives the job variety and makes it interesting. Anaesthetics is also known for its excellent and structured training. Trainees have senior support at all times of the day. It is also a very 'hands-on' specialty and involves many practical procedures such as lumbar punctures, arterial lines, tracheal intubation, and central venous line insertion.

As an F2, I had a 4 month post in anaesthesia and critical care. Whilst working on critical care, I attended daily consultant ward rounds and assisted with managing patients on the unit. Every day, I examined patients, analysed their blood results, and presented them to the consultant on duty. I was also on-call and attended emergencies and cardiac arrest calls. In theatre, I attended theatre and performed practical procedures such as tracheal intubation and central venous line insertion. I also completed my ALS certificate during this post.

I enjoyed my rotation and for that reason have chosen to apply for anaesthetics as an ST1.

Improved response

I have been interested in anaesthetics since medical school. As an undergraduate, I was very interested in human physiology; which is the foundation of anaesthetics. I am also quite a technophile and am interested in how new technology can be used to help patients. Anaesthetics has always been at the forefront of utilizing such innovations.

In my 4th year at medical school I was awarded a distinction for my 'special study module' in anaesthetics. I also won the MacGill Anaesthesia Prize awarded by the Royal Society of Medicine for an essay I wrote. In my final year at medical school, I applied to Foundation Year rotations that included an anaesthetics or critical care post.

During my 4 month post, I managed my own patients on the critical care unit. When on-call, I independently evaluated patients who were referred to our unit. I was taught many practical procedures and am now competent in endotracheal intubation and central venous line insertion. The DOPs for these procedures are in my portfolio. Later, I was responsible for my own theatre list with minimal supervision from my consultant. I also initiated and led an audit on hand-washing on the critical care unit. My findings were presented at our monthly departmental meeting.

I had the opportunity to speak to many consultants and trainees about anaesthetics as a career. I am aware that the training can involve long hours and at times be very stressful. However, I learnt so much in my F2 post and thoroughly enjoyed it. For this reason, I have chosen to pursue a career in anaesthesia.

I found my anaesthetics post to be a highly fulfilling job. I felt supported at all times but also had the opportunity to be challenged. I can think of no other specialty I would like to apply to more.

Positive indicators

- Has made an effort to learn about the specialty, e.g. talking to consultants, shadowed doctors in specialty, 'taster' week
- Aware of the pros and cons of·the job
- Has given significant thought to specialty choice
- Undergraduate prize, distinction, or merit in the specialty
- Gives coherent and logical reasons for applying
- Personality compatible with the specialty. For example, geriatrics: empathy, and communication skills.

In addition to the above, applicants to ST3+ posts should demonstrate:

- Participation in related projects such as presentations, research, publications, and courses.

- Prior experience in the specialty (but not more than 3 years as this may start counting against you).

Question 2

Can you tell me any disadvantages of a career in this specialty?

POSITIVE INDICATORS

- Displays insight into specialty
- Understands disadvantages of specialty
- Efforts made to find out about specialty
- Positive attitude

Question 3

What personal attributes make you suited for a career in this specialty?

POSITIVE INDICATORS

- Cites relevant personal attributes (see person specifications)
- Backs statement with specific scenarios or examples
- Relates relevance of attributes to specialty

Question 4

Why have you chosen this deanery?

POSITIVE INDICATORS

- Logical and coherent answer
- Shows interest in deanery
- Efforts made to research training programme
- Gives compelling professional and personal reasons

Audit and clinical governance

Question 1

Tell me about an audit you have participated in.

POOR RESPONSE

Last year, I participated in an audit on 'Falls in the elderly'. The purpose of the audit was to compare how elderly patients presenting with falls were being assessed by our department compared to NICE guidelines. The pro forma for data gathering was designed by ourselves. A list of elderly patients presenting with a fall over a 3 month period was generated by the audit department and their notes were requested. We went through all the notes retrospectively, checking for variables such as a full neurological examination, gait analysis, cognitive assessment and eyesight check.

The audit showed that patients were inadequately assessed after a fall and many did not have a detailed falls history or neurological assessment. The data were analysed and presented at our monthly departmental.

NOTE

This a poor answer and you would get a low score. It is impossible to ascertain the role of the interviewee in this audit. Talk about the role **you** played (not we) and describe the changes made as a result of the audit. Was there a re-audit or an attempt made to follow up at a later date? What will boost your score is listed below.

POSITIVE INDICATORS

- Initiated or designed audit
- Led or coordinated audit
- Presented at a meeting (particularly if national or regional)
- Changes in practice or protocol implemented
- Re-audit or attempt made to follow up

IMPROVED RESPONSE

Last year I participated in an audit about 'Falls in the elderly'. The purpose of the audit was to compare how elderly patients presenting with falls were being assessed by our department against NICE guidelines. It was a retrospective notes-based audit over a 3 month period. My role in the audit was to design a pro forma and gather and analyse data.

My analysis of the data showed that there were serious inadequacies. A third of patients did not have a detailed falls history. 20% of patients did not receive a full neurological examination. Nearly half of all patients did not have their gait or visual acuity assessed as per NICE guidelines.

I presented the findings at the Geriatric Department meeting followed by a teaching session to the junior doctors. I proposed the formation of a falls assessment pro forma which would ensure that patients would be assessed fully according to NICE guidelines. With my consultant I helped design a 'Falls in the elderly' pro forma which was introduced for use. The impact of these changes will be assessed in a re-audit which has been scheduled in a year's time. I offered my assistance in an advisory role.

Question 2

What is clinical governance and is it important for doctors?

NOTE

Resist the temptation to regurgitate a definition of clinical governance. Try to develop your own answer centred on your experiences of clinical governance. My suggestions include: critical incident reporting, audit, staff training, and continuous professional development. Before your interview, have a solid understanding of clinical governance. NHS Scotland has developed a useful education website, www.clinicalgovernance.scot.nhs.uk.

POSITIVE INDICATORS

- Demonstrates understanding of clinical governance
- Explains its importance for patient care
- Describes involvement in clinical governance
- Relates own experiences to improving patient care
- Gives coherent and logical explanations

Research and academic

Question 1

Why is it important for doctors to understand research?

POOR RESPONSE

Hundreds of clinical studies regarding novel treatments and procedures are published each week. In many specialties, the pace of change is rapid. For a clinician to provide the best care, understanding the research process is essential for them to critically appraise each paper. Understanding the evidence base for novel treatments will give it greater meaning to the doctor. This will also allow a better understanding of how new treatments are developed and ultimately improve patient care.

Understanding research also encourages a doctor to develop an inquisitive and questioning mind. This is important in the long term for future innovations and progress in clinical research.

Being involved in research also provides a doctor with a very useful set of generic skills. Research involves many disciplines; excellent and regular communication is often required. It trains doctors to improve their planning and organizational skills.

Note

The response above is good for an exam. For a job interview, it is poor; it fails to make the applicant stand out. A good response must show how **you** appreciate the importance of research, illustrated by **your own** research experience and related to **your** clinical practice.

Even if you have never directly participated in research, you could describe your experience of appraising papers, journal club participation, or searching the literature to answer a clinical question.

Good response

Last year, as part of my BSc research project, I was involved in stem cell research on cardiac myocytes. To design a study protocol, I learnt how to critically appraise hundreds of papers quickly. This has helped me as clinician as I regularly critically appraise papers. This has given me a better understand of the evidence base for new therapies. I can apply this evidence to each patient's individual circumstances and improve their care.

My research experience emphasized to me the importance of having a solid grounding in basic sciences in order to fully understand new therapies. I now regularly revise relevant physiology and basic sciences.

My project was complex and ambitious considering the time I was allocated. I had to plan the project carefully and be strict with my time management. Also, I had to be organized and work efficiently. This has improved my organizational and planning skills, which are essential for doctors.

Positive indicators

- Shows personal experience with research
- Uses personal experience to illustrate understanding
- Understands the purpose and impact of research
- Knows basic principles of research methodology
- Gives a coherent explanation for the importance of research

Question 2

Tell me about a paper you have read recently that has influenced you.

Note

This question has a dual purpose; your academic ability and interest in the specialty. As I advised in **CHAPTER 5 (PAGE 61)**, you need to be well-versed in a couple of research areas otherwise you could be throwing away easy interview points. When quoting a particular paper, remember the journal and the year and month in which it was published. Don't forget to relate the paper to the change in your clinical practice.

Positive indicators

- Critical analysis and awareness of different levels of evidence
- Applies evidence-based medicine
- Describes lessons learnt and change in practice
- Shows good understanding of papers and findings
- Demonstrates strong interest in specialty

Teaching

Question

What makes a good teacher?

Poor response

A poor teacher just teaches facts and often relies on didactic teaching. A good teacher engages the brains of students and encourages them to think for themselves. They achieve this by interactive teaching in small groups. Not only do students retain more information but they will be more interested in the subject.

Also, a good teacher adapts to the level of their students. For example, if teaching first year medical students, a good teacher would give a more basic talk than if he or she were teaching final year students.

Note

This candidate is not talking about him- or herself. The interview is about you! Talk about **your** experiences of teaching and how **you** use different techniques. If you have a formal teaching role, have organized a programme, or have attended a teaching course, use this chance to show off.

Maximize your interview score and sell yourself—I make no apologies for being repetitive!

Improved response

A good teacher engages the brains of students and encourages them to think for themselves. Last year, I was the teaching coordinator for third year medical students from Imperial College. I taught interactively as much as possible, in small groups. Rather than feeding facts, I frequently quizzed them and encouraged them to work out the answers from first principles. After each session, I summarized the main points and gave them handouts for revision purposes.

Although lectures would have been less time-consuming, students learn more with interactive teaching. I received excellent feedback from my students, which is contained in my portfolio here. Also, to be a good teacher, you need the right training. Last year, I attended a 'Teach the Teacher' course.

POSITIVE INDICATORS

- Uses different teaching methods, e.g. interactive, didactic
- Adapts to the level of experience of students
- Uses teaching aids, e.g. handouts, slides, photographs
- Has been trained in teaching methods
- Has positive feedback
- Has organized teaching locally or regionally

Question 2

Tell me about your experience of teaching.

POSITIVE INDICATORS

- Uses different teaching methods, e.g. interactive, didactic
- Uses teaching aids, e.g. handouts, slides, photographs
- Has designed or led a teaching programme
- Has formal training or has attended a course in teaching
- Has a formal teaching role
- Has had formal feedback on teaching

Leadership and teamwork

Question 1

Describe a situation when you worked as part of a team to help a patient.

GOOD RESPONSE

When I was an ST1 in geriatrics, we had Mrs Smith an 82-year-old admitted after a fall. She lived at home without any support. She had lost confidence and was struggling to regain mobility. We were concerned that she would require a residential home.

Her hearing aid was at home, making communication difficult. I contacted a neighbour who kindly brought it in. On examination, I found that she was significantly myopic. I had to arrange an escorted visit to a nearby optician. The PCT was initially unwilling to cover the cost of the spectacles as she was an inpatient. I was able to persuade them by reasoning that the spectacles were cost-effective, compared to residential home placement.

I reviewed all her medication and, where possible, minimized it. With her new glasses and hearing aid, her mobility started to improve noticeably. A few weeks later, she was ready for discharge.

NOTES

It is tempting to use an emergency scenario. But such scenarios are protocol-driven and are not the best for demonstrating your initiative or leadership. Choose the scenario you use at interview carefully, preferably in advance. The scenario needs to showcase **your** teamwork and leadership.

Talk about **your** delegation, decision making, and initiative. Describe how **you** overcame problems in detail. Compromising and negotiating are not signs of weakness; they show you can work with people with differing views. Do not make the mistake of describing a scenario without describing your contribution.

POSITIVE INDICATORS

- Participates in a non-confrontational way
- Negotiates, willing to compromise
- Shows leadership and delegates where appropriate
- Multiple disciplines or parties involved
- Considers others' ideas
- Shows initiative

Question 2

Tell me about a time you dealt with an underperforming colleague.

GOOD RESPONSE

As an ST1, I had a F1 doctor working in the team who was underperforming. He was constantly missing out vital tasks, forgetting to request important investigations, or get discharge summaries done on time. At the end of the day he often forgot to check blood results. His documentation was very poor and he would fail to write down the consultant's impression. This placed a great strain on the rest of team and the other junior doctors alienated him and were gossiping about him.

I made the point of talking to him in private, explaining the issues. I explored any difficulties he was facing and was as supportive and sympathetic as I could be. He admitted that he frequently did not understand what was going on during ward rounds as he was too focused on taking notes. He had simply forgotten many of the tasks he was meant to do.

I emphasized the importance of paying attention during the ward round, I showed him how he could improve his note-taking and save time by using standard abbreviations. I showed him how to keep a detailed 'tasks list' and advised him to complete his tasks in order of priority and urgency.

Later, there was noticeable improvement. I took the opportunity to praise him publicly on his progress. Throughout, I kept the consultant updated. At the end of his post, he received a satisfactory assessment. He also thanked me for all the support and advice, and left me with a 'thank you' card.

NOTE

There are many facets to this problem:

- Foremost is patient safety which you must address immediately.
- Second is to provide support and help to your colleague.
- If the problem is serious, you need to escalate it, either to a senior or through incident reporting.

You can adapt this approach for slightly different questions. For example, dealing with a drunk colleague or a colleague caught stealing.

POSITIVE INDICATORS

- Considers patient safety
- Is supportive and displays empathy with colleague
- Offers advice and practical support
- Uses initiative and displays problem solving ability
- Involves senior and other members of the team
- Critical incident reporting if indicated

Question 3

Describe a time when you were involved in a conflict at work? What was your role?

NOTE

You need to demonstrate your ability to listen, negotiate, and compromise. Choose the appropriate scenario in advance.

POSITIVE INDICATORS

- Explores and considers all sides involved
- Prioritizes patient care and safety
- Negotiates and discusses
- Involves others and seeks help
- Reflects on and learns from scenario

Question 4

Describe a time when you used your communication skills to help a patient.

Positive indicators

- Able to communicate with clarity
- Adapted style to suit the patient
- Able to listen and respond appropriately to the patient
- Minimizes jargon and explain any used
- Established a relationship of respect

Problem solving and decision making

You may be given a mock scenario to wrestle with at an interview station. This is slightly artificial as you are 'talking through' a scenario. The best way to prepare is to practise with a partner or with a small group of colleagues.

Question 1

Below is an exchange between an interviewer and a candidate. This is a mock problem-solving scenario. Learn from the model response of the candidate.

interviewer: You are the orthopaedic ST1. Mrs Gray, an 84-year-old woman, had a fall last week, fracturing her neck of femur. She had an uncomplicated hemi-arthroplasty and your registrar said that she could be discharged today. You have only seen the patient briefly on the ward round.

Mrs Gray's daughter is on the phone. She is unhappy about her mother being discharged. Please tell me what you would do next and the reasons behind your actions.

candidate: I would introduce myself and listen to the daughter's concerns. Ideally, I would try to arrange an appointment on the ward that day. I would gain verbal consent from the patient for me to discuss her case. Before the meeting, I would review the notes to refresh my memory and liaise with the nurses.

I would meet Mrs Gray's daughter in a private room and ask a colleague to hold my bleep to minimize interruptions. I would explore the daughter's concerns in full and as is reasonable, would try to address her concerns. I would make a complete record of the discussion in the case notes later.

interviewer: The daughter thinks that her mother is confused, which is new for her. She is worried about her mother's safety as she lives alone without support. What next?

CANDIDATE: I would reassess Mrs Gray including a Mini-Mental State Examination. I would also seek the opinion of the nurses, physiotherapist, and other staff involved with her care.

INTERVIEWER: Mrs Gray's MMSE is 14/30. The nurses report that she was very forgetful and has a tendency to wander about the ward inappropriately. The physiotherapist thinks her mobility is good, but she needs prompting with each task. What now?

CANDIDATE: Discharge would be unsafe. I would perform a full neurological examination and request a confusion screen such as a chest X-ray, urinalysis, and blood tests. I would update the nurses and my seniors of the confusion and change in plan. Mrs Gray's daughter would have to be kept informed too and I would provide her with my contact details for the future.

INTERVIEWER: Your registrar is on the phone. He insists that Mrs Gray can still be discharged today. What do you do now and why?

CANDIDATE: I don't think it is safe to discharge her and her new confusion needs investigation. I would reiterate these concerns to my registrar and insist she is unsafe for discharge. I would also update my consultant.

POSITIVE INDICATORS

- **Patient safety**: Mrs Gray appears to be significantly confused. You have to postpone discharge. Your concern for Mrs Gray's safety must override your registrar's orders. Blind obedience to seniors can be dangerous.
- **Listens**: Being able to listen to the family, patient, nurses, and other members of the multidisciplinary team is essential.
- **Communication**: Keep all parties updated including relatives, ward staff, and other doctors.
- **Decision making and initiative**: Re-evaluating the patient is often a good idea. Show that you can act independently by instituting investigation and treatment.
- **Patient confidentiality**: If the patient has capacity, obtain consent to discuss their case with relatives.

Question 2

Mr Rich, an 88-year-old man, is an inpatient under your care. He presented with generalized abdominal pain. A CT of his abdomen reveals he has probable colorectal carcinoma with multiple liver and bone metastases. Mr Rich's daughter has been told of the diagnosis. She is adamant that her father should not be informed of his diagnosis and is threatening legal action if this is disclosed. What would you do next?

POSITIVE INDICATORS

- Explores daughter's concerns and reasons
- Handles matter with sensitivity and concern
- Attempts to determine Mr Rich's capacity and mental state
- Respect patient's autonomy
- If appropriate, involves other specialties, e.g. psychiatry
- Involves seniors and other colleagues

Question 3

Pretend I am a patient who needs to have a colonoscopy. Explain the procedure to me.

- Makes an introduction and explains role
- Minimizes jargon, uses everyday language
- Gives a clear, easily understood explanation
- Explains reasons and complications
- Has a warm and approachable manner

Coping with pressure

Question 1

You are the medical ST3 on night shift. An F2 is the other member of your team. You are managing a patient with a life-threatening exacerbation of asthma on the ward. Your F2 calls you urgently. A patient on another ward has been fitting for 5 minutes. Rectal diazepam has not worked. Please explain what you would do next and your reasoning.

POSITIVE INDICATORS

- Willing to call for help from seniors and other specialties, e.g. anaesthetics, consultant
- Finds out more about the patient
- Considers distance from ward
- Gives telephone advice, if appropriate
- Considers needs of both patients
- Has rational approach to scenario

You then get a call from the coronary care unit. A patient who is post-myocardial infarction has just gone into ventricular tachycardia. What will you do next?

POSITIVE INDICATORS

- Finds out more about the patient, e.g. blood pressure, responsiveness
- Gives telephone advice, if appropriate
- Delegates and involves other colleagues
- Considers the needs of all patients

Question 2

Tell me about a stressful situation at work and how you dealt with it.

POSITIVE INDICATORS

- Prioritizes tasks
- Is flexible and adapts to dynamic situations
- Has a logical and sensible approach to problems
- Delegates work and involves other colleagues
- Involves seniors

Question 3

What do you do to relax when you are not working?

NOTE

You need to demonstrate means of dealing with stress. Don't come across as being obsessive about work. Talk about hobbies, sport, socializing, or even spending time with your family. If you de-stress by getting blasted at the pub then keep this quiet!

POSITIVE INDICATORS

- Demonstrates the ability to deal with stress
- Has appropriate mechanisms
- Recognizes the need for managing stress

Empathy and sensitivity

Question 1

Describe a situation in which you used empathy or sensitivity to make a difference to a patient.

GOOD RESPONSE

Mrs White, an elderly woman, had been admitted with recurrent falls. She lived at home without support. On the ward, she was refusing physiotherapy, citing tiredness. At the MDT meeting, we were concerned and residential home placement was being considered. This saddened me, as it was an option I knew she was desperate to avoid.

I would talk to Mrs White everyday and got to know her. Gradually, I developed a rapport and gained her trust. She had lost confidence since falling and she was terrified of falling at home with nobody around to rescue her.

Also, she had pain in her right groin but had not told anybody as she didn't want to create a fuss. I requested a pelvic X-ray and this showed a pubic ramus fracture. I prescribed her regular analgesia. Everyday, I would review Mrs White's pain and continually encourage her with her physiotherapy. I reassured her that she would be fully supervised.

Mrs White's mobility improved substantially and she soon could walk with a frame. Before going home, side rails were fitted at her home and she was given a pendant alarm. Before she left, Mrs White thanked me for all I had done and even gave me a bottle of whisky.

POSITIVE INDICATORS

- Listens to patient's concerns and develops rapport
- Detects subtle cues
- Demonstrates warmth and concern
- Creates a trusting atmosphere
- Attempts to resolve the problem by responding to needs

Question 2

Describe a situation when you displayed empathy or sensitivity to a colleague.

POSITIVE INDICATORS

- Prioritizes patient safety
- Listens to colleague's concerns
- Detects subtle cues
- Demonstrates warmth and concern
- Attempts to resolve the problem by responding to needs

Professional integrity

Question 1

Tell me about a time when you made a mistake. What did you do next? How did your mistake affect your work afterwards?

Good response

> As an F1, I had a patient who was diagnosed with a hospital acquired pneumonia. My registrar instructed me to prescribe intravenous Tazocin. His drug chart stated he was penicillin allergic. I did not know that the generic name of Tazocin was piperacillin and that it was actually a penicillin, so I prescribed it. Fortunately, the pharmacist noticed my error soon after.

> My first concern was the patient's safety and I immediately informed the nurses of my error. Fortunately, none of the antibiotic had been administered. I immediately informed my registrar and consultant of the error. When I had the chance, I apologized to the patient for the error that nearly took place and explained that it was because I had failed to look up. Instead of being angry, he thanked me for my honesty. Later, I completed a clinical incident reporting form so that the 'near-miss' could be recorded by the Trust.

> Immediately after that incident, I the read up on the commonly used antibiotics. From then on, I made it a point to look up the side effects and cautions of every drug I prescribed, particularly if it was something that I was unfamiliar with. I also tend to double check any allergies by asking the patient or checking the 'allergy band'.

Notes

Nobody likes talking about their mistakes, especially at a job interview. But everybody makes mistakes and the interviewers understand this. The purpose of this question is to determine if you can learn from them and change your practice. Also, you have to show concern for patient safety and escalate the error (see Positive indicators).

Choose the scenario to use at interview in advance and with care. Avoid mistakes that resulted in death or serious injury. Also avoid errors that were due to your negligence.

Positive indicators

- Patient safety: makes this a top priority and takes immediate action if required.
- Reflects and learns: shows ability to learn from the mistake. Has taken action and changed practice as a result of the error.

- Probity: is honest and open to the patient. Explains and apologizes to the patient (or family) promptly.
- Escalation: informs seniors or consultant of error and subsequent action.
- Clinical governance: critical incidence reporting.

REFERENCES

1 Guidance for Applicants, National (England and Wales) Selection 2010, Interview Process and Scoring System. Royal College of Paediatrics and Child Health, London (www.rcpch.ac.uk).

2 Academic Clinical Fellow Specimen Interview Evaluation Form. 2010 National Institute for Health Research Trainees Coordinating Centre, Leeds (www.nihrtcc.nhs.uk).

3 Good Practice Toolkit, Phase 3: Selection Centre Guidance. Joint Committee on Surgical Training, London (www.jcst.org).

CHAPTER 7

The specialties

The advice given in this chapter is specialty specific and is supplementary to other chapters. It is important to refer back to the rest of the book. The competition ratios quoted are from the MMC website (www.mmc.nhs.uk).

General Practice (GP)

General practitioners; masters in no system, specialists in their patients. In 2009, there were approximately two applicants per post. Statistically, this is the least competitive specialty. Nevertheless, GPs won't let just anybody join their ranks. To secure a training post you must sit a computer-based test and attend a selection centre.

Arguably, GP has the most organized and forward-thinking selection process. It managed to steer clear of the MMC debacle which plagued other specialties in 2007. Specialties such as CMT and Anaesthetics are trying to emulate the GP selection process.

Career development

Unlike other specialties, you don't have to demonstrate your commitment. There is no need to 'boost' your CV with publications, research projects, and presentations as these are not considered at selection. Nevertheless, before committing yourself to a lifelong career, it would be advisable to get a feel for it beforehand. Shadow a GP or organize a 'taster'. A 4-month post in GP would be even better.

The selection process

The selection process is split into three stages.

STAGE 1: LONG-LISTING

If the essential criteria are fulfilled, you automatically proceed to stage 2. It consists of completing an online application form and is relatively straightforward. There is no 'white space' you need to fill in to promote yourself.

STAGE 2: SHORT-LISTING

The real competition begins here. Applicants have to sit two different types of questions under exam conditions; Clinical Problem Solving and Professional Dilemmas (situational judgement test). Applicants are short-listed solely on the basis of their test score. **CHAPTER 4, PAGE 47** has advice on acing such selection exams.

STAGE 3

The selection centre is the final hurdle. The Royal College of General Practitioners (RCGP) has done away with interviews as they was found to have little discriminatory value. Instead, applicants sit two types of assessments:

- written exercise
- simulation exercise (role-playing scenario)

Perform well in these exercises and the job is yours. In **CHAPTER 5** I provide advice on these forms of assessment.

Broadly speaking, applicants are assessed in five domains:

- communication skills
- professional integrity
- empathy and sympathy
- problem solving
- coping with pressure

You can get a feel for the marking scheme from a paper published by the *British Journal of General Practice* in 2000.[1] The first author, Fiona Patterson was involved in developing the selection process for GP. At the time of writing (2010) she was the assessment and psychometric adviser to the RCGP.

In the paper there is a table of competencies and behavioural observations. The marking scheme for stage 3 is likely to be based on this. If you are applying to general practice, I strongly recommend reading this paper online (free).

Paper which shaped the GP selection process

'The model could be employed for future research in design of selection techniques for the role of GP' [*British Journal of General Practice* (2000), **50**, 188–193]

SHOULD I JOIN A COURSE?

There are dozens of businesses offering help to prospective applicants, for a fee. Most are commercial and you must shop carefully.

Some businesses offer to 'check' your application form at stage 1. The application form is straightforward and in plain English. Save your money and follow the instructions on the form!

To do well at the stage 2, I recommend practising lots of questions. There are numerous books and websites you can join to access these. Make sure the practice questions closely resemble the actual exam.

A course would be most beneficial for stage 3. It isn't essential, and many applicants have been successful without attending a single course. However, if you are weak in a particular area or want a confidence boost, than a quality course will help.

> GP: a course would be most beneficial for stage 3

Below is a list of businesses (in alphabetical order) that have been recommended by previous applicants and have established reputations:

- Apply2Medicine: www.apply2medicine.co.uk
- EMedica: www.emedica.co.uk
- ISC Medical: www.medical-interviews.co.uk
- Pastest: www.pastest.co.uk

REFERENCE

1 Patterson, F. et al. (2000). A competency model for general practice: implications for selection, training, and development. British Journal of General Practice, **50** 188–193.

Core Medical Training (CMT)

After General Practice, this is the specialty with the most applicants. With nine applicants per post (in 2008) it is one of the less competitive specialties.

The application process

Application is online via a single process for all applicants in England and Wales. Applicants are allowed to state their top three deaneries. Short-listing is done nationally and the highest-ranked candidates will be interviewed by the deanery of their choice. Interviews are organized locally but follow a standardized format and marking scheme.

Career development

GETTING AHEAD

- Pass the MRCP. Completing part 1 or 2 demonstrates your commitment.
- Publish a case report or original articles.
- Present at regional and national conferences.
- Work towards a medical specialty early on.

COURSES

- ALS
- Teach the teacher

PRIZES AND PRESENTATIONS

- Royal Society of Medicine (RSM): the Alan Edwards prize is awarded for the best case presentation. There are additional awards in different medical specialties. The RSM website (www.rsm.ac.uk) contains all the details.
- RCP (London): awards elective bursaries to medical students. Teale essay prize for trainee doctors.
- Read other medical specialties in this chapter. Many have prizes and presentation opportunities for medical students and trainees.

JOURNALS

- *BMJ Case Reports* publishes a very high volume of case reports each month.
- *Geriatric Medicine* accepts review articles.
- *British Journal of Hospital Medicine* accepts reviews and case reports from trainees.
- *West London Medical Journal*: not very well-known, but it is calling for original articles and case reports.

Interviews

Recent interviews have consisted of three stations each lasting 10 minutes:

- Station 1: role-playing scenario
- Station 2: clinical and problem solving scenarios
- Station 3: portfolio, clinical governance, commitment to specialty

COMMON INTERVIEW QUESTIONS

- Tell me about an interesting audit? Tell me about a paper you've read that's changed your clinical practice?
- Is understanding research important for clinicians?
- Questions on work-based assessments—you may be asked for your opinion on them.
- Why have you chosen CMT?
- Where do you see yourself in 5–10 years' time?

CLINICAL SCENARIOS

QUESTION 1

A 55-year-old alcoholic with known oesophageal varices presents with frank haematemesis and melaena. He is tachycardic but normotensive. Haemoglobin is 8 g/dL (previously 12 g/dL).How would you manage this patient?

Positive indicators:

- Resuscitate, i.e. large-bore IV access, fluids, cross-match blood
- Be aware of Rockall score
- Urgent endoscopy
- Consider antibiotics, glypressin, Sengstaken–Blakemore tube
- Inform seniors, consider critical care
- Consider prophylactic propanolol, TIPSS (transjugular intrahepatic portosystemic shunt)
- Alcohol cessation and offer rehabilitation (later, when recovering)

QUESTION 2

A 70-year-old smoker with COPD (chronic obstructive pulmonary disease) has just been admitted with severe breathlessness, wheeze, and cough with green sputum. He is talking in incomplete sentences through his oxygen mask with a respiratory rate of 18 breaths/min. On auscultation, he has reduced air entry and marked expiratory wheeze throughout.

His arterial blood gas results are:

FiO_2: 0.75
pH: 7.35
pCO_2: 6.8 kPa
pO_2: 21.1 kPa
Base excess: 4.9 mmol/L

What do the these blood results suggest? How would you manage him?

Positive indicators:

- Identify compensated respiratory acidosis
- Recommend controlled oxygen
- Nebulizers, antibiotics, steroids, if appropriate; theophylline
- Reassess regularly
- Consider NIV (non-invasive ventilation) or ITU early on
- Later; smoking cessation, consider home oxygen

Suggestion: Revise your arterial blood gases and the BTS (British Thoracic Society) guidelines on managing asthma and COPD. Be aware of the indications for NIV.

QUESTION 3

A 55-year-old man has been admitted with a severe, 'sharp' epigastric pain present for several hours. His blood pressure is 88/45 mmHg and he is tachycardic. He appears pale and cool to the touch. On examination, there is epigastric tenderness and voluntary guarding but the rest of his abdomen is soft. What are your differential diagnosis and how would you manage him?

Positive indicators:

- Formulate a reasonable list of differentials
- Resuscitate patient, i.e. I.V. fluids
- Investigations including blood results, glucose, ECG, and chest X-ray
- Involve seniors and surgeons (second opinion)
- Consider CT imaging if stabilized

Suggestion: Do not jump straight into requesting a CT. You must always stabilize your patient first. An acute abdomen is not always due to a surgical cause. Differential diagnoses include aortic dissection, myocardial infarction, diabetic ketoacidosis, pancreatitis, perforated oesophagus, cholecystitis, ischaemic bowel.

QUESTION 4

A 26-year-old man is an inpatient who first presented with diabetic ketoacidosis. He was very unwell on arrival a few days ago but appears to have improved. An arterial blood gas shows he is no longer acidotic. He is currently on an insulin infusion with a blood sugar of 14 mmol/L. He is eating and drinking and wants to go home.

He tells you that he wants to go home that evening for his daughter's birthday. He is adamant he is leaving and would self-discharge if need be. Your registrar is on a holiday and the consultant is in an important meeting. What would you do?

Positive indicators:

- The patient is well and is not acidotic; he does not need any I.V. insulin.
- Patient education on type 1 diabetes mellitus:
  - *recognition and treatment of a hypoglycaemic episode.*

- *aware of need to return if vomits or is unwell*
- *has contact number of a diabetes nurse*
- He should be taught use of a glucometer and insulin pens.
- Outpatient follow-up arranged

QUESTION 5

Management of an unconscious patient. Go to **ANAESTHESIA, CLINICAL SCENARIO 1, PAGE 125**.

QUESTION 6

Pneumothorax; management and guidelines. Go to **RESPIRATORY, CLINICAL SCENARIO 3, PAGE 182**.

PROBLEM SOLVING SCENARIOS

QUESTION 1

An 89-year-old woman had a cerebrovascular accident. Despite 3 weeks of care on the stroke unit, she has shown little signs of recovery. She has not regained consciousness and her GCS is persistently 7/15. She has been fed via nasogastric tube. Her family want to take her home. They have heard about feeding via a PEG tube and want to talk to you about it. What would you do next?

Positive indicators:

- Communicate openly with family
- Explain poor prognosis and quality of life
- If the patient has no capacity, the doctor has to decide for the patient, with their best interests in mind (not their family)
- Discuss options, i.e. withholding active treatment, withhold feeds

QUESTION 2

Dealing with difficult colleague at work. Read **LEADERSHIP AND TEAMWORK, QUESTION 2, PAGE 99**.

ROLE-PLAYING SCENARIOS

QUESTION 1

Consent a patient for thrombolysis. Go to **EMERGENCY MEDICINE, ROLE-PLAYING SCENARIO 1, PAGE 132**.

QUESTION 2

Explain a diagnosis to an anxious patient. Go to **CARDIOLOGY, ROLE-PLAYING SCENARIO 1, PAGE 170**.

QUESTION 3

Speak to a concerned relative. Go to **CARE OF THE ELDERLY, SITUATIONAL SCENARIO 2, PAGE 172**.

QUESTION 4

Patient education to an asthmatic with poor compliance. Go to **RESPIRATORY, ROLE-PLAYING SCENARIO 1, PAGE 181**.

QUESTION 5

Explain to a patient with suspected pulmonary embolus the need for admission. Go to **RESPIRATORY, ROLE-PLAYING SCENARIO 2, PAGE 182**.

TOPICAL QUESTIONS

- Hospital-acquired infections, e.g. MRSA, *Clostridium difficile*
- Obesity in medicine: how to tackle this growing problem?

Acute Common Care Stem (ACCS)

For many trainees, this is the gateway to Acute Medicine, Emergency Medicine, or Anaesthetics. At 19 applicants per post, ACCS is competitive compared with other specialties at CT1. At the time of writing (2010) recruitment was local, although national recruitment is being considered.

The specialty has been piloting the use of selection exams (i.e. clinical problem solving and situational judgement tests). So far, the feedback has been good. Future applicants should expect selection to incorporate such tests. **CHAPTER 4** has more on selection exams.

Career development

ACCS is a stepping-stone to one of the acute specialties. For career development, read the relevant specialty in this chapter.

Interviews

Previous interviews have consisted of a three-station interview with one clinical scenario. Read the advice and practice the scenarios for all of the three specialties. There will be a strong slant towards the specialty theme of the post; focus on it.

The South-West Deanery has piloted a selection centre consisting of: structured interview, portfolio station, presentation, clinical simulation, and two role-playing scenarios. This may become the future interview format.

Common interview questions

- Define probity. Give me examples of a doctor's behaviour not meeting an appropriate standard.
- Tell me about the last paper you read.
- Tell me about an audit you did.

Situational scenario

QUESTION 1

Coping with multiple casualties in the Emergency Department. Go to **EMERGENCY MEDICINE, SITUATIONAL SCENARIO 1, PAGE 131**.

QUESTION 2

Dealing with a dodgy consultant. Go to **SECTION 7.10, SITUATIONAL SCENARIO 2 121**.

Clinical scenarios

QUESTION 1

You are asked to review a 60-year-old patient in A&E with breathlessness. He is diaphoretic, tachycardic, tachypnoeic, and has saturations of 80% on air. What are your immediate management priorities?

QUESTION 2

A 45-year-old patient on the medical admission unit just had an episode of haematemesis. He looks pale and is tachycardic but normotensive. Tell me how you would manage him.

QUESTION 3 (CT2)

You are anaesthetizing an otherwise well ASA 1 (American Society of Anesthesiologists classification 1, normal healthy patient) for a minor surgical procedure when you notice their saturations on the monitor falling rapidly. What action do you take?

QUESTION 4

Management of variceal bleeding. Go to **CORE MEDICAL TRAINING, CLINICAL SCENARIO 1, PAGE 113**.

QUESTION 5

Management of severe exacerbation of COPD. Go to **CORE MEDICAL TRAINING, CLINICAL SCENARIO 2, PAGE 113**.

QUESTION 6

Management of a hypotensive patient with epigastric pain. Go to **CORE MEDICAL TRAINING, CLINICAL SCENARIO 3, PAGE 114**.

QUESTION 7

Management of an unresponsive patient and role-playing. Go to **ANAESTHESIA, CLINICAL SCENARIO 1, PAGE 125**.

QUESTION 8

Dilemma in theatre. Go to **ANAESTHESIA, CLINICAL SCENARIO 2, PAGE 126**.

QUESTION 9

Pneumothorax management. Go to **RESPIRATORY, CLINICAL SCENARIO 3, PAGE 182**.

ROLE-PLAYING SCENARIOS

QUESTION 1

Explain general anaesthesia to a patient. Go to **ANAESTHESIA, ROLE-PLAYING SCENARIO 1, PAGE 126**.

QUESTION 2

Explain a cancelled procedure to an angry patient. Go to **ANAESTHESIA, ROLE PLAYING SCENARIO 2, PAGE 126**.

QUESTION 3

Talk to a pre-operative patient with an abnormal ECG. Go to **ANAESTHESIA, DATA INTERPRETATION SCENARIO 1, PAGE 127**.

QUESTION 4

Consent a patient for thrombolysis. Go to **EMERGENCY MEDICINE, ROLE-PLAYING SCENARIO 1, PAGE 132**.

TOPICAL QUESTIONS

- What do you think of the 4-hour rule in the Emergency Department?
- The evolving role of the specialty Acute Medicine
- Do you know anything about new working patterns in Anaesthesia?
- There is an increasing call for consultants to be present out-of-hours. What do you think of this?
- What do you think of routine ultrasound guidance for central venous line insertion?

Surgery in General (CT1 and CT2)

In 2008, there were 12 applicants per post. This is undoubtedly one of the more competitive specialties and is oversubscribed. This could get worse in the next several years as a reduction in training posts is expected.[1] There is also a severe bottleneck downstream at ST3. Many trainees have struggled for years to get into a training post.

Career development

You should concentrate on developing your CV as early as possible. Try to plan for two stages ahead. For example, a medical student should plan for CT1, an F1 should plan for ST3, an ST3 for a consultant post!

HOW TO GET THE EDGE

- Get published in a surgical journal
- Present at surgical conferences
- Complete an audit
- Complete the MRCS
- Participate in your medical school's surgical association (students)

COURSES

In previous years, each course attended from the list below would secure you a point at short-listing:

- Basic Surgical Skills Course
- Care of the Critically Ill Surgical Patient
- ATLS (Advanced Trauma Life Support)
- ALS (Advanced Life Support)
- Train the Trainer course

PRIZES AND PRESENTATIONS

Medical students:

- Association of Surgeons in Training (ASiT): medical student prize, elective bursaries
- Royal College of Surgeons (RCSeng): Preiskel Elective Prize, Professor Harold Ellis Prize

Junior doctors:

- ASiT: their annual conference accepts a large number of posters for presentation and is well worth a go. There is also a short paper presentation and prize
- Royal Society of Medicine: Adrian Tanner Prize (case report and presentation)
- Association of Surgeons of Great Britain (ASGBI): their International Surgical Congress has an opportunity to present and win prizes. More competitive but prestigious
- RCSeng: awards a few research fellowships annually

PUBLICATIONS

- *Annals of The Royal College of Surgeons of England*: accepts case reports, research, articles and review. Definitely worth submitting to if you have a reasonable article. Peer-reviewed and widely recognized.
- *Bulletin of The Royal College of Surgeons of England*: accepts articles for the 'trainee's forum'. Peer-reviewed.
- If you present at the ASiT conference, your abstract is automatically published.
- *BMJ case reports*

PRACTICAL PROCEDURES

It isn't essential to have a logbook of surgical procedures. However, keeping a log of all the procedures you have assisted in will demonstrate your interest and diligence. Definitely recommended.

Application process

At the time of writing (2010) recruitment is organized by individual deaneries. A national recruitment process is being considered but no definite plans have been announced.[1] Each deanery's application forms and interview processes are different. However, if you are not geographically fussy, applying to as many deaneries as you can will maximize your chances of success.

Interviews

In recent years many deaneries in have had a three-station format:

- portfolio & verification station
- structured interview: audit and clinical governance, motivational question, research
- clinical or role-playing scenario

Only a few deaneries have had a practical skills station.

PORTFOLIO STATION

Some deaneries use this as a verification station. Bring evidence for **everything** listed in your application form. Keep your portfolio organized so it is easy to access. Read the portfolio section in **CHAPTER 3 (PAGE 27)**.

ROLE-PLAYING SCENARIOS

The scenarios will be similar to those in the MRCS viva. The section 'Problem solving and decision making' in **CHAPTER 6, PAGE 101** has additional role-playing scenarios to practice.

QUESTION 1

You might be asked to consent a patient for a procedure relevant to your specialty. For example, lipoma removal, colonoscopy, incision and drainage of an abscess.

Positive indicators:

- Explains common and serious complications
- Explains reasons for procedure
- Gives time for questions and checking understanding
- Reassuring and friendly demeanour
- Uses everyday language, minimizes jargon

QUESTION 2

Explain a procedure to a patient (actor). The actor may be instructed to be very nervous and have underlying concerns.

Positive indicators:

- As for Role-playing scenario Question 1

QUESTION 3

Talk to an angry pre-operative patient. Go to **ANAESTHESIA, ROLE-PLAYING SCENARIO 2, PAGE 126**.

QUESTION 4

A conversation with a grumpy radiologist. Go to **TRAUMA AND ORTHOPAEDICS, ROLE-PLAYING SCENARIO 1, PAGE 154**.

CLINICAL SCENARIOS

The clinical scenario is commonly a trauma call or an emergency on the surgical wards. Also, be prepared for a medical emergency that commonly affects surgical patients, such as a pulmonary embolus or myocardial infarction. Revise your ATLS manual. Read the 'Clinical scenarios' section in **CHAPTER 6 (PAGE 71)** for more advice on clinical scenarios.

QUESTION 1

You are the CT1 on-call. A 35-year-old man involved in a road traffic accident (RTA) is in the Emergency Department. He has pain and bruising in the left upper quadrant. Your registrar is scrubbed up in theatre. Tell me what you would do next.

Positive indicators:

- Systematic approach as in ATLS
- Resuscitation: large-bore intravenous access, cross-match, fluids
- Recognizes potentially life-threatening injury, i.e. ruptured spleen.

- Involves consultant or second on-call
- Informs theatre, involves anaesthetist

Whilst dealing with your first patient, a nurse on the surgical ward calls you urgently. A patient has significant haematemesis. The ward is 15 minutes walk away.

Positive indicators:

- Gets relevant information over phone, i.e. observations, past medical history
- Prioritizes based on severity of patient illness
- Gives telephone advice to ward
- Balances needs of different patients appropriately
- Ask for help from other specialties, i.e. Casualty registrar, medical registrar

QUESTION 2

A 57-year-old man involved in a RTA is brought in to A&E. He has a significant degloving injury of his right hand with cold and pale digits and an unpalpable radial pulse. How would you manage this patient? How long is the critical ischemia period?

Positive indicators:

- Similar to Clinical scenario Question 1

QUESTION 3

Management of an acute abdomen. Go to **CORE MEDICAL TRAINING, CLINICAL SCENARIO 3, PAGE 114**.

QUESTION 4

An unconscious patient on the ward. Go to **ANAESTHESIA, CLINICAL SCENARIO 1, PAGE 125**.

QUESTION 5

An elderly patient with a hip fracture. Go to **TRAUMA AND ORTHOPAEDICS, CLINICAL SCENARIO 1, PAGE 154**.

QUESTION 6

Managing a trauma call on your own. Go to **TRAUMA AND ORTHOPAEDICS, CLINICAL SCENARIO 2, PAGE 155**.

PRACTICAL ASSESSMENTS

A few deaneries have practical stations such as suturing a laceration or excising a skin lesion. This is covered in the section 'Practical skills assessment' in **CHAPTER 5 (PAGE 68)**.

- The European Working Time Directive (EWTD): do you think it good for surgical trainees?
- How would you determine if a patient is competent to consent?
- Do you think whistle-blowing should be encouraged? Explain.

Sources of information

- Royal College of Surgeons of England (RCSeng): www.rcseng.ac.uk
- The Association of Surgeons in Training (ASiT): www.asit.org
- Association of Surgeons of Great Britain and Ireland (ASGBI): www.asgbi.org.uk

REFERENCE

1 Presentation entitled 'Medical Specialty Training 2010' by Alison Carr, Dean Advisor, MMC England. Presentation hosted at: www.foundationprogramme.nhs.uk

Anaesthesia

Depending on the deanery, there were 4 to 10 applicants per post in 2009. This makes anaesthetics one of the less competitive specialties.

The application process

By 2011, recruitment to CT1 and ST3 in England and Wales will be national through a single website. Individual deaneries will still be running interviews along nationally agreed guidelines.

In 2008–2010, the Royal College of Anaesthetists (RCOA) piloted selection exams (situational judgment and clinical problem solving tests) as part of short-listing. These pilots have confirmed the validity of formal assessments.[1] It is increasingly likely that selection exams will be part of the selection procedure in future (see CHAPTER 4, PAGE 47).

Career development

COURSES

To maximize your score you should attend at least four of the courses in Group 1 below and as many of the courses as you can in Group 2.[2]

Group 1:

- ALS (Advanced Life Support)
- ILS (Immediate Life Support)
- BASICS (British Association for Intermediate Care courses)
- IMPACT (Ill Medical Patients' Acute Care And Treatment)
- Local critical care course
- Airway course
- Simulator course (e.g. Emergency Anaesthetic Simulation Exercise Course)

Group 2:

- ATLS (Advanced Trauma Life Support)
- APLS (Advanced Paediatric Life Support)
- EPLS (European Paediatric Life Support)
- Regional simulator
- Royal College or National Airway courses

PRIZES

Medical students

- RCOA: President's Award for Undergraduate Research (or audit)
- RSM (Royal Society of Medicine): essay prize, elective bursaries
- The Association of Anaesthetists of Great Britain and Ireland (AAGBI): Wylie Medal Undergraduate (essay) Prize, elective funding
- The Intensive Care Society (ICS): essay prize

Junior doctors

- RCOA: the Maurice P. Hudson Prize
- AAGBI: the Anaesthesia History (essay) Prize, GAT Audit Prize
- ICS: State of the Art (research and audit) Prize

PRESENTATIONS

- RSM: essay prize
- Obstetric Anaesthetists Association (OAA): annual meeting (oral and poster)

- ICS: annual spring meeting
- AAGBI: annual scientific meeting
- British Pain Society (BPS): annual meeting
- Difficult Airway Society (DAS) annual meeting

PUBLICATIONS

- *Anaesthesia News:* accepts case reports and letters to the editor. It is also an excellent means of keeping abreast of issues
- *Bulletin of the Royal College of Anaesthetists:* accepts letters and original articles.
- *CPD Anaesthesia:* accepts reviews and multiple choice questions (MCQs)

Interviews

The usual format has been three stations:

Station 1: portfolio. Show evidence of the following:
- *Work-based assessments*
- *Reflective practice*
- *Personal development plan*
- *Relevant audit/project work*
- *Logbook of procedures carried out (it is a good idea to log all procedures from an early stage to demonstrate competencies)*
- *Courses and teaching*
- *ST3: Obstetric Anaesthesia and Intensive Care Medicine competencies, Basic Level Training Certificate, logbook.*

Station 2: talk through the following:
- *situational scenario and/or*
- *data interpretation*

Station 3: role-playing scenario
- *See the section 'Role-playing scenario' in* **CHAPTER 5 (PAGE 71)** *for practice scenarios*

CLINICAL SCENARIOS

QUESTION 1 (CT1)

You are asked to review a patient (actor) on the ward. There will be an observations and drug chart. The patient is unresponsive and snoring heavily. Talk through your actions and present the case to an anaesthetist who arrives.

Positive indicators:

- Assesses patient systematically, Airway, Breathing, Circulation, Disability (GCS), Examination, Glucose.
- Formulates a logical plan, e.g. maintains airway (chin lift or Guedel), gives oxygen, calls for help early, establishes IV access, considers naloxone, investigations, e.g. CT brain.
- Scrutinizes observations and drug chart, e.g. low respiratory rate, opiates, benzodiazepines.
- Presents case clearly and effectively to the anaesthetist.

QUESTION 2 (ST3)

You are the Anaesthetic ST3 managing an elective list by yourself in theatre. The list is already 45 minutes behind and the surgeon is urging you to 'crack on'. Your next patient is a 50-year-old man with no major co-morbidities. On laryngoscopy, the patient has a grade 4 Cormack view. How would you proceed? Your consultant has not responded to his pager.

Positive indicators:

- Seeks additional assistance or involves another consultant
- Considers options, e.g. fibre-optic intubation, awake intubation under local anaesthesia
- Understands potential risks and takes appropriate action
- Able to explain rationale clearly

ROLE-PLAYING SCENARIOS

QUESTION 1 (CT1)

You are the Anaesthetic CT1. Mrs Brown is a 68-year-old woman awaiting an elective laparoscopic cholecystectomy later that day. You are to visit her on the ward and take an anaesthetic history pertinent to the procedure. Explain to her the general anaesthetic and answer any concerns that she may have.

[**Actor instructions**: No previous illness, no regular medication. You are allergic to penicillin; it gives you a wheeze and a rash. You are terrified of having a general anaesthetic. 25 years ago, your father had an elective hip replacement. The anaesthetic did not wear off for many hours and he had to be ventilated on the intensive care unit. But you don't want to create a fuss and won't mention it unless the doctor gives you an opportunity to.]

QUESTION 2 (CT1)

Mr Thompson is due to have a elective knee replacement today. However, you notice that he was pyrexial this morning and, on examination, has bronchial breathing on one side. A chest X-ray confirms consolidation. You are to inform Mr Thompson that his procedure is being postponed and the reasons for this.

[**Actor instructions**: You have been waiting for your knee replacement for 4 months. Your operation has already been postponed once because of a staffing issue. You are fed up and get angry when informed of the cancellation. You assume that the cancellation is due to poor organization.]

DATA INTERPRETATION

QUESTION 1

You are shown a pre-operative ECG of a young man undergoing elective arthroscopy. Interpret the ECG [complete heart block] and talk through your actions.

Positive indicators:

- Correctly interprets the ECG
- Recognizes potential risk, i.e. peri-operative bradycardia, asystole
- Consults cardiologist for advice and consideration of pacing
- Reconsiders options, e.g. postpones procedure, involves patient

QUESTION 2

You might be given an arterial blood gas to interpret. Potential scenarios could include:

- An asthmatic patient with hypoxia and respiratory acidosis.
- A COPD patient with respiratory acidosis and markedly raised pO_2.
- An unresponsive patient with metabolic acidosis, e.g. diabetic ketoacidosis (DKA), overdose.

Remember to interpret the results with the clinical history. Revise arterial gas interpretation and be prepared to talk through the management of common emergencies.

TOPICAL QUESTIONS

- Nurse anaesthetists; what do you think of them? Are you in favour of their increasing number?
- Tell me about sugammadex. Do you know of situations when it might be advantageous over suxamethonium?
- Could be asked about any recent NICE guideline pertinent to anaesthesia, e.g. 2010 VTE prophylaxis, Matching Michigan. Guidelines can be found on the AAGBI (www.aagbi.org), NICE (www.nice.org.uk), and National Patient Safety Agency (NPSA; www.npsa.nhs.uk) websites.

Sources of information

RCOA: www.rcoa.ac.uk
AAGBI: www.aagbi.org

ICS: www.ics.ac.uk
BPS: www.britishpainsociety.org
DAS: www.das.uk.com

REFERENCES

1 Anderson et al. Selection to Anaesthesia and Acute Care Common Stem Core Training Programmes in the South West of England. Accepted for Anaesthetic Research Society Winter Meeting; 2009 Dec; London.

2 CT2–ST3 Shortlisting Score Criteria (2010). Royal College of Anaesthetists, London.

Emergency Medicine (ST4)

This section covers entry into ST4 Emergency Medicine. ACCS is covered in a separate section (**PAGE 116**).

Most trainees are expected to enter at CT1 (ACCS). On completion of core training (CT3), trainees have to compete for a higher specialist training post in Emergency Medicine (ST4). Recruitment is national, organized by the College of Emergency Medicine (CEM).

Career development

MEDICAL STUDENTS

- Volunteer to help out in the Major Incident Medical Management and Support (MIMMS) Course as a 'demonstrated body'. You get to be covered in fake blood and it shows your enthusiasm for the specialty. Contact your local coordinator.
- Get involved with the emergency medicine society in your medical school.
- RSM: Emergency Medicine Students' (essay) Prize.

COURSES

ALS, ATLS, and APLS are compulsory for ST4. Additional courses, particularly ultrasound and airway courses will help at short-listing.

- Ultrasound courses: Emergency Ultrasound Course, Handheld Echocardiography for Critical Care, Basic Echocardiography for Acute Management

- Airway courses: SATS (Severn Airway Training Society) Difficult Airway Course, UK Training in Emergency Airway Management Course
- Major Incident Medical Management and Support Course
- Teaching courses

PRIZES AND PRESENTATIONS

- CEM Autumn Conference: a large number of poster (over 100) and oral presentations are accepted for this conference each year. The Roderick Little Prize is awarded for the best trainee presentation.
- RSM: Emergency Medicine (research and presentation) Prize

CLINICAL EXPERIENCE

Experience in other specialties is a plus—specifically, Cardiology, Geriatrics, Respiratory, Obstetrics and Gynaecology, or a surgical specialty.

HOW TO GET THE EDGE

- Pass the Membership of the College of Emergency Medicine (MCEM) part A
- Do a good audit
- Present at the CEM conference
- Attend the courses above
- Publish

Interviews

INTERVIEW FORMAT

In previous years, the ST4 interviews have followed a seven-station format.[1]

1. Portfolio and specialty-specific questions. There is an emphasis on topical issues and motivation in applying for Emergency Medicine
2. Clinical scenario
3. Situational (problem solving) scenario
4. Notes-based assessment
5. Role-playing scenario, e.g. a complaining patient.
6. Teaching station, e.g. teach a junior doctor.
7. Pilot station which did not count towards selection. Evaluate another doctor completing a workplace-based assessment.

COMMON INTERVIEW QUESTIONS

- Why do you want to do Emergency Medicine?
- Why have you applied to this deanery?

- Can you tell me of a time when you made a mistake, and tell me what you did about it?
- What makes you angry in relation to Emergency Medicine?
- Tell me about your strengths and weakness.

TOPICAL QUESTIONS

- The 4-hour target: do you think it has improved patient care? Know why and when it was implemented. Be prepared to discuss its strengths and weaknesses. If you take a viewpoint, be prepared to justify it.
- Consultants being present during out-of-hours. This is the current gold standard, but will have implications for consultant working hours and training numbers. Be able to discuss the issue at depth.

CLINICAL SCENARIOS

CHAPTER 5 (PAGE 71) covers resuscitation scenarios. You may have a mock scenario, similar to ALS or ATLS. Below are some scenarios that have cropped up in the past.

QUESTION 1

Variceal bleeder. Go to **CORE MEDICAL TRAINING, CLINICAL SCENARIO 1, PAGE 113**.

QUESTION 2

Severely hypoxic patient. Go to **CORE MEDICAL TRAINING, CLINICAL SCENARIO 2, PAGE 113**.

QUESTION 3

An acute abdomen. Go to **CORE MEDICAL TRAINING, CLINICAL SCENARIO 3, PAGE 114**.

QUESTION 4

Trauma call. Go to **SURGERY IN GENERAL, CLINICAL SCENARIO 1, PAGE 121**.

QUESTION 5

Deal with an uncooperative patient. Go to **PSYCHIATRY, CLINICAL SCENARIO 1, PAGE 144**.

QUESTION 6

Primary pneumothorax. Go to **RESPIRATORY, CLINICAL SCENARIO 3, PAGE 182**.

SITUATIONAL SCENARIO

Below is a sample scenario.

You are on night duty for the Emergency Department. The only other doctor in the department is a CT1 (SHO). It has been a quiet night, no patients are waiting. Suddenly, a nurse bursts in: two cases have just been brought in by ambulance:

- Case 1: 20-year-old man from a high-speed motorcycle accident. Open tibial fracture, possible rib fractures. Tachycardic but normotensive. SaO_2 is 99% on air with a respiratory rate of 18 breaths/min. He is screaming in agony and his right leg is dressed and soaked in blood.
- Case 2: 5-year-old boy with breathlessness. Tachycardic but normotensive. SaO_2 is 94% on high-flow O_2. Respiratory rate is 14 breaths/min. He is drowsy but rousable.

What do you do next? Which case will you attend to first and why?

Positive indicators:

- Calls for urgent help: fast bleep paediatrics and surgeons
- Delegates: directs CT1 colleague and nurses
- Recognizes the sickest patient. The 5-year-old boy needs your attention first. He is exhausted and probably peri-arrest
- Rapid assessment and resuscitation

QUESTION IB (CONTINUED FROM QUESTION IA)

The paediatric registrar is dealing with an arrest on the ward. The surgeon is scrubbed up in theatre. Your consultant is driving in, but he will not arrive for 20 minutes.

Positive indicators:

- Consider alternatives, e.g. paediatric consultant, anaesthetist, critical care consultant
- Ongoing resuscitation

QUESTION IC

Another patient arrives by blue light ambulance. It is a 50-year-old man found on the street unresponsive and pulseless by a bystander. He is in PEA (pulseless electrical activity) arrest and has had 30 minutes' CPR in total. The paramedics have intubated and administered IV adrenaline and atropine with no effect. Core temperature of 36°C.

Positive indicators:

- Urgent call to medical registrar or anaesthetist
- Considers the needs of all three patients and balances them appropriately
- Recognises that the prognosis is very poor after 30 minutes of PEA arrest
- Does not abandon other two patients

NOTES-BASED ASSESSMENT

You might be asked to review a set of clinical notes and identify safety issues. Be prepared to propose a plan and changes. Remember patient identifiers, date, time, appropriate units.

ROLE-PLAYING SCENARIOS

QUESTION 1

Explain to and consent a patient for thrombolysis of an ST elevation myocardial infarction. [The actor could be very anxious and might want to know the exact risk of haemorrhage.]

Suggestion: Read up about the risks and contraindications of thrombolysis in the *Oxford Handbook of Clinical Medicine*. It is a pressurized situation, but you need to explain that, on average, they are better off with thrombolysis. Give time for questions and use everyday language.

QUESTION 2

Deal with the complaint of a patient whose tooth was chipped when having an oropharyngeal airway inserted in the Emergency Department for coma secondary to alcohol consumption. [The actor might be instructed to be rude and angry.]

Suggestion: No matter how tempting it is to be rude back to this sort of patient, don't! Always remain polite and non-confrontational. (See **CHAPTER 6, PAGE 101** for more role-playing scenarios.)

QUESTION 3

A reluctant patient with suspected PE (pulmonary embolism). Go to **RESPIRATORY, ROLE-PLAYING SCENARIO 2, PAGE 182**.

TEACHING STATION

This is used to evaluate your communication skills and ability to teach. For example, teach a third-year medical student how to read an ECG. You might have 2 minutes to prepare and 5 minutes to teach. At the start, check the student's prior knowledge and at the end outline how to take the learning further, e.g. practise interpreting more ECGs.

REFERENCE

1 Advice to applicants applying for specialty training in Emergency Medicine at specialty training year 4 (Higher Specialty Training) in 2009. CEM, London (www.collemergencymed.ac.uk).

Obstetrics and Gynaecology

In the last decade, the number of UK graduates applying to Obstetrics and Gynaecology has dropped to 'dangerously low' levels.[1] The Royal College of Obstetricians and Gynaecologists (RCOG) is strongly encouraging more UK graduates to apply. In 2008, there were 6 applicants per ST1 post, making it one of the less competitive specialties.

Career development

PRIZES

Medical students:

- RCOG: elective awards, Special Study Module (SSM) Prize, Tim Chard Case History Prize, Richard Johanson Obstetric (research) Prize.
- Wellbeing of Women: medical student elective bursaries
- British Maternal and Fetal Medicine Society: research or audit prizes
- RSM: Dame Josephine Barnes (essay) Award

FY and ST:

- RCOG: Herbert Erik Reiss Memorial Case History Prize
- British Maternal and Fetal Medicine Society

PRESENTATIONS

- British Maternal and Fetal Medicine Society Annual Conference (oral and poster)
- RSM: Herbert Reiss Trainees Prize (oral and poster)
- British International Congress of Obstetrics and Gynaecology
- Regional Meetings: check deanery websites and e-mail administrators for dates

EXAMS: FY AND ST

- MRCOG Part 1: recommended for ST1 applicants but compulsory for ST3

COURSES: FY AND ST

- Advanced Life Support Training in Obstetrics
- Basic Surgical Skills Course, RCOG
- Advanced Life Support in Obstetrics (ALSO)

Application process

Obstetrics and Gynaecology training is run-through and most trainees enter at ST1 though there are entry points at ST2 and ST3. The application form is online and short-listing is organized nationally (England and Wales). Short-listing in 2009 evaluated the following areas:[2] communication, problem solving and initiative, research and publications.

Interviews

Interviews are held locally by deaneries and follow a nationally agreed three-station format:

- Portfolio and interview
- Clinical scenario
- Role-playing scenario

PORTFOLIO AND INTERVIEW STATION

- Give me examples of reflective practice.
- Evidence from Mini-Clinical Evaluation Exercise (Mini-CEX), case-based discussion (CBD) and Direct Observation of Procedural Skills (DOPS)
- Tell me about an audit you have participated in.
- Why do you want to do Obstetrics and Gynaecology?
- Give an example of a clinical incident that has changed your practice.

ROLE-PLAYING SCENARIO

CHAPTER 5 has more on role-playing scenarios.

CLINICAL SCENARIOS

QUESTION 1

As an F1, you're called to see a patient 1 day post-hysterectomy. She is hypertensive and tachycardic. On examination you find her abdomen rigid with guarding and rebound tenderness. Your registrar is 'scrubbed up' in theatre with an emergency Caesarean section and cannot respond. What do you do next?

Positive indicators:

- ABC, resuscitate, analgesia
- Investigate: repeat bloods, arterial blood gas, erect chest X-ray (urgent)
- Escalate to consultant or second on-call
- Prepare for theatre: group and save, alert theatres, involve anaesthetist

You call the consultant on-call, a locum. He asks you to consent the patient for an exploratory laparotomy. Whilst on the phone, the patient's husband arrives. He is very angry. What do you tell the consultant? How would you deal with the patient's husband?

Positive indicators:

- As an F1 you don't have the experience to consent for a laparotomy: **be firm** with the consultant.
- Know your limitations
- Allow the husband to express his feelings. Listen and explore concerns
- Apologize and be sympathetic

Maintain a calm and professional demeanour

QUESTION 2

Rank these five scenarios in order of priority. Explain what you would do and your reasoning behind your decisions:

- 45-year-old with previous endometriosis presenting with umbilical pain radiating to the right iliac fossa
- 50-year-old, 1 day post-hysterectomy hypertensive and tachycardic
- Elderly patient with calf pain, recently been diagnosed with advanced ovarian cancer.
- Pregnant woman, 30 weeks, with clots and large, fresh vaginal bleeding
- Referral from the medical registrar regarding a 65-year-old woman with post-menopausal bleeding

Suggestion: It is important that you explain your rationale when you prioritize—almost as if you were talking through the scenario. **CHAPTER 5** has more advice on prioritization exercises.

QUESTION 3

You are the ST1 for Obstetrics and Gynaecology and have been asked to review a 30-year-old in the Emergency Department. She has been taking Microgynon (combined oral contraceptive pill) for 6 years. Last week, her left calf started swelling and becoming painful. What do you think it could be and what would you do next?

Positive indicators:

- DVT (deep vein thrombosis) main concern
- Investigate, bloods, ultrasound Doppler
- Cover with treatment dose heparin
- If DVT confirmed, stop Microgynon and consider contraception
- Thromboprophylaxis for long-haul flights, stay hydrated

TOPICAL QUESTIONS

- What is the effect of the European Working Time Directive on Obstetrics and Gynaecology trainees?

- How can we encourage junior doctors to train in Obstetrics and Gynaecology?
- Be ready for questions on recent publications on maternal and child health, e.g. Saving Mothers' Lives.
- Be familiar with guidelines on the management of obesity in pregnancy (ST2–ST4)
- CEMACH (Confidential Enquiry into Maternal and Child Health), CEMD (Confidential Enquiry into Maternal Deaths)

Sources of information

RCOG: www.rcog.org.uk

British Maternal and Fetal Medicine Society: www.bmfms.org.uk

Centre for Maternal and Child Enquiries: www.cmace.org.uk

TWOGs Trainees in Wales Obstetric and Gynaecology Society: www.wales.nhs.uk

REFERENCES

1 Improving Recruitment to Obstetrics and Gynaecology. Report of a joint working party of the RCOG and AAOG. December 2006 (www.rcog.org.uk/files/rcog-corp/uploaded-files/WPRImprovingRecruitment2006.pdf).

2 Short-listing Score Sheet, Specialty Training in Obstetrics and Gynaecology ST1–ST2. RCOG 2009.

Radiology

Recruitment is hosted by a single deanery (England and Wales). Entry is at ST1 and training is run-through. Interviews may still be organized by individual deaneries.

Career development

HOW TO GET AHEAD

- Join the societies listed below in 'Prizes and presentations' and participate in meetings.
- 'Shadow' in the Radiology Department. 'Tasters' are handy for this.

Courses

- Radiology-courses.com (Northwick Park Hospital, London) runs several different courses suitable for junior doctors, e.g. the A&E Radiology Survival Course and the Chest X-ray Survival Course.

Prizes and presentations

- Royal College of Radiologists: essay prize and elective bursaries for students. The annual meeting is a chance for doctors to present audits, cases, and research with the chance to win prizes
- British Institute of Radiology: fellowship for student electives
- UK Radiological Congress: opportunities to present cases and posters
- Society of Radiologists in Training (SRT): hosts annual meeting with posters

Publications

- *Clinical Radiology* and the *British Journal of Radiology* are well known, but most case reports are difficult to get published.
- *Eurorad*: has a peer-reviewed online pictorial or case report archive. Published by the European Society of Radiology

Many medical and surgical journals have a dedicated 'images' section:

- *BMJ*: Minerva
- *Heart*: Images in cardiology
- *Thorax*: Images in thorax
- *Archives of Surgery*: Images of the month

Interviews

A common format is three interviews each lasting 10 minutes:

- Station 1: portfolio, audit, and achievements
- Station 2: situational scenario, teamwork, professionalism
- Station 3: aspirations, commitment to the specialty, understanding of specialty

Common interview questions

- Why do you want to do radiology?
- What makes a good radiologist?
- How do you think your previous experience would help you in a career in radiology?
- Tell us about a case you have been involved in where radiology was central to your patient's management.

Role-playing scenarios

You are informed by a radiology nurse that a colleague of yours is about to start doing an ultrasound-guided drainage procedure but she suspects your colleague is under the influence of alcohol. What would you do?

Positive indicators:

- Patient safety: postpone procedure or find alternative operator
- Colleague safety: find private place to rest, ask nurse to monitor
- Escalate: inform clinical director, another consultant
- Personal: offer support, talk to colleague

Data interpretation

Some applicants have been asked to report on a variety of images. Be systematic. Check the patient details followed by the radiological investigation. Don't blurt out the most obvious abnormality—there may be more than one.

Give a list of your differentials with the most likely one first. Interpret the images in the context of the clinical story. For example, a chest X-ray shows bilateral hilar lymph node enlargement. If the patient is an elderly Asian patient with night sweats and a purulent cough, tuberculosis should be considered first. If it were a 30-year-old man born in the UK, with no known TB contact, sarcoidosis should be considered.

There may be multiple possible diagnoses (as in the example above) and it is important to mention them in your answer in order of likelihood. If appropriate, recommend a plan, e.g. respiratory physician referral or next imaging modality.

Other examples include:

- Barium swallow study showing oesophageal tumour
- MRI of the female pelvis showing multiple fibroids
- CT of the head showing an acute subdural haemorrhage

Clinical scenario

QUESTION I

You are the Radiology Registrar on-call. Almost simultaneously, you get urgent requests for four different patients:

- Patient 1: CT chest and abdomen for patient post-road traffic accident (RTA). Haemodynamically unstable. FAST scan shows free fluid around the spleen.
- Patient 2: CT (head to pelvis) for patient post-high-speed RTA. Haemodynamically stable.

- Patient 3: CT brain for an elderly man with a 2-hour history of right-sided hemiparesis. Suspected stroke.
- Patient 4: CTPA for known metastatic pancreatic cancer and now hypoxic and peri-arrest.

How would you prioritize these patients? Explain your reasoning.

Suggestion: Your answer will depend on local policy and available resources. Consider the following:

- Patient 1: needs resuscitation first—not imaging!
- Patient 2: urgent CT required.
- Patient 3: potential for thrombolysis, depending on local policy. CT brain is relatively quick. Urgent CT would be most appropriate.
- Patient 4: this patient could have a cardiac arrest in the scanner! Has the medical registrar reviewed the resuscitation status?

QUESTION 2

You have been asked to asses a patient in CT urgently. The patient has become breathless and appears blotchy immediately after having contrast.

Suggestion: Know the common acute medical problems which may happen in the Radiology Department, such as above. Other examples would include contrast extravasation, post-nephrostomy or percutaneous transhepatic cholangiography (PTC) sepsis.

TOPICAL QUESTIONS

- Increasingly, non-radiologists are involved in image interpretation or interventional work. For example, specialist radiographers now interpret images. Will there still be a need for radiologists in the future?
- Radiology is becoming increasingly specialized around organ systems. For example, there is sub-specialization in musculoskeletal, genitourinary tract, and neuroradiology. Do you think this is a good idea? Please explain.
- What do you think of outsourcing radiology work such as chest X-ray interpretation overseas? Explain your reasoning.

Further reading

Royal College of Radiologists: www.rcr.ac.uk
Society of Radiologists in Training : www.thesrt.org.uk

Paediatrics and Child Health

In 2009, there were four applicants for every post in Paediatrics and Child Health. Paediatrics is thought to be significantly undersubscribed.[1] Recruitment is via a national online application system (England and Wales). The interviews are organized locally following nationally agreed guidelines. Training is run-through with entry points at ST1 to ST4.

Career development

MEDICAL STUDENTS

- Enter for the essay competitions hosted by the RCPCH (Royal College of Paediatrics and Child Health)
- Apply for a bursary to attend the RCPCH Annual Spring Conference
- Do extra-curricular work with children, e.g. summer camp, children's charities

FY DOCTOR

- Present at meetings, e.g. RSM and Paediatric Scottish Society meetings
- Pass 1a or 1b of the MRCPCH exam (Member of the RCPCH)
- Attend the RCPCH Spring Conference or Paediatric Scottish Society Summer Meeting

Get certified in APLS (Advanced Paediatric Life Support) or NLS (Newborn Life Support)

Interview format

In recent years a carousel of three stations, each 10 minutes in duration, has been used. Below is a mock format:

- Station 1: role-playing scenario
- Station 2: presentation station
- Station 3: structured interview

SPECIALTY QUESTIONS

QUESTION I

What did you do during medical school to find out about a career in Paediatrics?

Suggestions:

- Work experience, e.g. summer schools, babysitting
- Voluntary work
- Electives, Special Study Modules
- Paediatric societies in medical school

QUESTION 2

What attracted you to Paediatrics?

QUESTION 3

What qualities make you suited to Paediatrics?

ROLE-PLAYING SCENARIOS (COMMUNICATION SKILLS)

QUESTION I

A 16-year-old boy presenting with fever and photophobia is suspected to have viral meningitis. He needs to have a lumbar puncture to confirm or exclude it. Your task is to explain the procedure to him and the reasons for doing it. [The teenager thinks he only has the flu. He is terrified of needles.]

Suggestions:

- Adapt your style to communicating to a teenager
- Avoid jargon
- Remember to listen, i.e. needle phobia
- Explain the importance of excluding or diagnosing meningitis

QUESTION 2

A 10-month-old baby with severe pneumonia had the wrong blood samples taken (by a colleague). You are to inform the child's father of this and explain the need for a repeat blood test. [The 'child's father' has been instructed to be furious and distrustful of doctors.]

Suggestions:

- Apologize and shows sensitivity
- Calm, reassuring and professional manner
- Explain importance of blood tests
- Listen and explore concerns

CLINICAL SCENARIOS

Revise common conditions and emergencies in the specialty. Even if stuck, answer in a structured way: resuscitation, focused history and examination, investigation and treatment:

- How would you manage a 5-year-old child with a fever in the Emergency Department?
- How would you manage a 16-year-old with severe exacerbation of asthma?
- How would you manage a 3-month-old baby with pyrexia in the Emergency Department? (ST3)

- Describe what 'failure to thrive' is and how you would investigate. (ST3)
- How would you manage a neonate who had an unresponsive episode a few hours after birth? (ST3)

TOPICAL ISSUES

- The impact of the European Working Time Directive (EWTD) on Paediatric training
- The implications of having so many females in Paediatrics
- Child protection and the role of doctors

PRESENTATION TOPICS

- How to reduce alcohol consumption in teenagers
- Paediatrics is not just medicine for smaller people
- Preventing childhood obesity

There are some more tips and suggestions in **CHAPTER 5 (PAGE 70)**.

REFERENCE

1 Presentation entitled 'Medical Specialty Training 2010' by Alison Carr, Dean Advisor, MMC England. Presentation hosted at: www.foundationprogramme.nhs.uk

Psychiatry

If you are a UK graduate the Royal College of Psychiatrists (RCPsych) will be keen to recruit you. There is a severe shortage of UK graduates applying.[1] With nine applicants per post, Psychiatry is one of the relatively less competitive specialties.

Career development

MEDICAL STUDENTS

The RCPsych are really keen to attract students:

- Prizes and bursaries: there are fantastic opportunities for your CV and wallet. There are bursaries for electives, research, and attending meetings. The RCPsych even awards essay prizes for each sub-specialty.
- Enrol as a Student Associate of the RCPsych. This is free and entitles you to attend the Student Associate Conference and Summer School (week-long).

Both are bonuses to your CV. Meals are provided and for Summer School, accommodation is provided.

- Voluntary work related to psychiatry, e.g. learning disability, dementia day centre.

FY DOCTOR

- Enrol as a Student Associate of the RCPsych. You may get co-opted to being student or FY representative on the Trainee Committee.
- Get published: the *Student Associate Newsletter* and *The Psychiatrist* (peer-reviewed) are published by the RCPsych. As a student or trainee doctor you have a reasonable chance of getting published. E-mail the respective editors with your article ideas.
- Attend and present: each faculty of the RCPsych organizes its own annual conferences. There is usually a call for posters, abstracts, or audits. Presenting at a national conference would place you ahead of the competition.
- Organize a taster week for yourself.

Application process

There are two main entry levels are at CT1 and ST4. Recruitment for CT1 (England) is via a national recruitment campaign coordinated by the Royal College of Psychiatrists. There are plans for this to extend to ST4 in 2011.[2]

The breakdown of short-list scoring in 2010 was as follows: commitment to specialty (22%), audit (14%), publication or research (14%), presentations (14%).[3]

Interview

FORMAT (CT1)

Previous applicants describe a three-station process, with each station lasting 10 minutes.[4] Below is a sample carousel based on their descriptions:

- Station 1: audit question, research question, clinical scenario
- Station 2: teaching question, coping with pressure question, profession-alism question, situational scenario
- Station 3: (1) Portfolio. There was a focus was on mini-PAT (mini-Peer Assessment Tool) and reflective practice. Other work-based assessments were also reviewed. (2) Pre-interview task. Applicants were given 20 minutes to write a summary of their portfolio and achievements. Write neatly and be structured! Don't forget to display your 'outstanding points' (SEE THE SECTION ON 'BACKGROUND QUESTIONS' IN CHAPTER 6, PAGE 84).

Specialty questions

- Describe the features and management of depression.
- What are the features, causes, investigations, and management of delirium?
- How would you assess a psychotic patient?
- Who is allowed to access a patient's notes?

Situational questions (CT1)

Question 1

You are the ST1 on-call. There are two patients waiting to be seen: (1) a 25-year-old woman with a deliberate overdose of seven paracetamol tablets she took 2 hours ago and (2) an agitated, delirious 80-year-old man on a medical ward who is trying to leave:

- Who will you see first and why?
- The elderly man is delirious and hallucinating. Tell me how you will assess and manage him.
- How would you assess the 25-year-old woman? How would you evaluate her suicide risk?

Suggestion: The scenario is deliberately ambiguous with minimal information. In many cases there is no right answer. You need to show that you can prioritize appropriately. The 80-year-old man will be at risk if he leaves the ward. Unless security is present, he may 'escape' soon. Consumption of seven paracetamol tablets is usually not fatal. Also, you need to wait 4 hours before you can request a blood test for levels.

Question 2

What would you do if you suspected your consultant was becoming psychiatrically unwell?

Suggestions:

- Ensure patient safety
- Ensure consultant safety
- Involve another consultant or clinical director
- Contact Occupational Health or the 'Practitioner Health Programme'

Clinical scenarios (CT1)

Question 1

What would you do if asked to assess a patient in the Emergency Department who was refusing to speak at all?

Suggestions:

- Involve someone the patient trusts to try and explain and encourage communication.
- Observation to assess mood and signs of psychosis.
- Collateral history from relatives, police, paramedics.
- Physical examination (e.g. catatonic signs) and blood tests.
- Personal safety, e.g. alarm buttons, joint assessment, positioning near exit.

QUESTION 2

A 60-year-old man has taken a paracetamol overdose. How would you assess his suicide risk?

QUESTION 3

An intravenous drug user has been an inpatient for 2 days. He is insisting that you increase his dose of methadone. What would you do and why?

QUESTION 4

An inpatient with bipolar disorder was admitted voluntarily. Later that week, she demands to see you wanting to self-discharge. What would you do next?

TOPICAL ISSUES

- The Mental Capacity Act 2005 and its application. In 2007, Kerrie Wooltorton took an overdose of anti-freeze. She had an advance directive and was deemed to have capacity. Treatment was not commenced and she later died. This case generated much discussion and controversy
- The Mental Health Act (2007) and how it relates to patients with severe personality disorder
- Assisted Dying for the Terminally Ill Bill
- European Working Time Directive
- The recruitment shortage in psychiatry

REFERENCES

1 Robert Howard, Dean of the Royal College of Psychiatrists in an interview with Channel 4, broadcast 4 June 2009 (www.channel4.com/news/article.jsp?id=3190557).

2 Dr Val Yeung, *Newsletter*, Trent Division RCPsych, July 2009 (www.docstoc.com/docs/34255698/Newsletter—Trent).

3 Royal College of Psychiatrists (2010). Shortlisting framework for scoring Core Training Level 1 (CT1) application forms (www.rcpsych.ac.uk/PDF/Shortlisting%20framework%202010.pdf).

4 Josie Jenkinson, Top Tips for the CT1 Interviews, *Student Associate Newsletter*, February 2010 (www.rcpsych.ac.uk/training/studentassociates/newsletters/newsletterfebruary2010.aspx#5).

Public Health

In 2008 there were six applicants per post making Public Health one of the less competitive specialties.[1] Nevertheless, the Faculty of Public Health (FPH) won't accept just anyone to specialize in the 'bigger picture'. First, you have to complete an online application form and enter a national recruitment process. You then have to pass two psychometric tests (verbal and numerical reasoning) before being offered an interview. The interview process is unique and is described further in this section.

Career development

HOW TO GET THE EDGE

- Pass the MFPH, Part A
- 'Taster' experience
- Relevant courses
- Attend and present at public health meetings
- Relevant research and publications

PRIZES AND PRESENTATIONS

Medical students:

- RSM: Brooke Elective Bursary
- FPH: Sir John Brotherston (essay or research) Prize, Cochrane Prize (elective or research)

Junior doctor:

- Present your poster at the FPH's annual conference.
- UK Public Health Association Public Health Forum: an opportunity to present at an international conference. In 2009, hundreds of posters were presented

COURSES

- Statistics
- Evidence-based medicine
- Critical appraisal of papers

PUBLICATIONS

- BMC *Public Health* is an online, peer-reviewed journal. On the plus side it publishes a large number of research articles (over 50 a month), so you stand a better chance of getting published. The downside is that there is a 'processing charge' of approximately £1100.
- *Critical Public Health*
- *Journal of Public Health*: research and original articles.
- *PH.com* is the newsletter of the FPH: submit article your ideas to the editor.

Interviews

INTERVIEW FORMAT

Interviews are standardized nationally with the same questions and marking scheme. In recent years, interviews have consisted of the following:

- Interview (four stations): including two problem solving tasks (12 minutes each)
- Presentation station (30 minutes for preparation)
- Observed, group exercise (50 minutes)

COMMON INTERVIEW QUESTIONS

- What experience in your work, related to public health, has motivated you to pursue a career in public health?
- Give an example of a situation in your work where there were difficulties working with other team members. How did you address this and what would you do differently next time?

PROBLEM-SOLVING SCENARIO

QUESTION I

Recent figures from Emergency Departments across the county demonstrate a recent surge in the number of cyclists injured in road traffic accidents. How would you investigate this and what action you would suggest?

Suggestions:

- Consult all 'stakeholders', i.e. Emergency Department, cyclists, local council, schools, motorist associations, cycling groups
- Attempt to identify causes for upsurge, e.g. more cyclists, increased traffic density
- Corroborate this with data from other sources, e.g. police, insurance companies
- Suggest reasonable plan, e.g. speed cameras, cyclist education
- Re-evaluate changes

Previous applicants have been asked to critically appraise a paper. They have also been asked if they would adopt a new initiative on the basis of the paper. This is an exercise in evidence-based medicine (EBM). Make sure you know about EBM, which is at the heart of public health.

PRESENTATION STATION

Previous applicants have had to give a 4-minute presentation on a public health matter such as obesity, smoking, or pollution. There was time to prepare beforehand and acetates were provided. Be well-read in a few public health issues. Read the section on 'Presentation station' in **CHAPTER 5 (PAGE 70)** for advice on presentation.

GROUP EXERCISE

Four applicants go through an observed exercise together. There is a trained assessor for each applicant. Applicants are given 20 minutes to prepare followed by a 30-minute group discussion. An example of a group exercise is given below.

You are the public health representatives for McBunbury, a large town. Below are four different public health initiatives which have been proposed. You are to go through the pros and cons of each initiative. Which initiative will benefit the town the most? You will have to decide which initiative you choose to bid for funding.

- Free or subsidized sports equipment for schools. TIKE, a major sports equipment manufacturer, has offered to sponsor this initiative for 1 year. No public funds are required for the first year.
- Public smoking ban. Subject to approval from the town council. It would impose a ban on smoking in all public places such as bus stops, train stations, parks, and streets.
- Chlamydia screening programme. To be offered to those under 25 in schools, colleges and university.
- Childhood obesity: an educational programme aimed at parents. It teaches parents about childhood obesity, healthy eating, and exercise.

The section on 'Group discussion' in **CHAPTER 5 (PAGE 77)** has more on group exercises.

TOPICAL QUESTIONS

The FPH regularly publishes statements and toolkits. I recommend reading some of them so you are able to discuss the issues in detail (available from the FPH website, www.fphm.org.uk).

- 12 steps to better public health—a manifesto (http://www.fph.org.uk/uploads/manifesto_public_health.pdf)
- The health needs of asylum seekers (www.fph.org.uk/uploads/bs_aslym_seeker_health.pdf)

- Healthy weight, healthy lives: a toolkit for developing local strategies (www.fph.org.uk/healthy_weight,_healthy_lives%3A_a_toolkit_for_developing_local_strategies)
- Position statement on fat (www.fph.org.uk/uploads/ps_fat.pdf)
- Alcohol and public health (www.fph.org.uk/uploads/ps_alcohol.pdf)

REFERENCE

1 Foundation Doctor Advisory Board, 18 November 2009. UK Foundation Programme Office.

General Surgery (ST3)

Competition is fierce with 19 applicants per post in 2008. Unfortunately, this is anticipated to get worse. A reduction in training posts is anticipated in the next few years. For surgery as a whole there are more CCT holders than there are consultant posts.[1]

Career development

There is a bottleneck getting into ST3 and you're going to have to work hard on building your portfolio. The selectors are looking for applicants who have taken part in research and have publications and presentations at conferences. Unsuccessful applicants will have a better chance when they reapply with a PhD, MD, or research fellowship.

HOW TO GET THE EDGE

- Be first author in multiple peer-reviewed journals
- Present at regional or international conferences
- Research, i.e. PhD, MD, research fellowships
- MRCS

RESEARCH

Officially, research is not compulsory. But many trainees are of the opinion that an MD or MSc is essential to get into training. There are tailored MScs which can be done full or part time. University College London, Imperial College, and Cardiff University are just some of the institutions that offer this.

COURSES

Same as for Surgery in General (CT1) **(PAGE 118)**.

PRIZES AND PRESENTATIONS

Same as for Surgery in General (CT1) **(PAGE 118)**.

PUBLICATIONS

Same as for Surgery in General (CT1) **(PAGE 118)**.

Interviews

Typically, this follows a five-station format:

- Role-playing scenario (communication skills)
- Portfolio and interview
- Clinical and management scenarios
- Situational scenario (leadership and teamwork)
- Practical skills

ROLE-PLAYING SCENARIOS

See the section on 'Problem solving and decision making' in **CHAPTER 6 (PAGE 101)** for more advice and scenarios.

QUESTION 1

Consent a patient [actor] for an appendicectomy.

Positive indicators:

- Explain common and serious complications
- Explains reasons for procedure
- Gives time for questions and checks understanding
- Reassuring and friendly demeanour
- Uses everyday language, minimizes jargon

QUESTION 2

Talk to an angry pre-operative patient. (See **ANAESTHESIA, ROLE-PLAYING SCENARIO 2, PAGE 126**).

PORTFOLIO STATION

Your portfolio will be scrutinized. It helps if you have the following:

- Surgical DOPS (at least three)
- Multiple procedure-based assessments (at least three)
- Logbook with significant experience

CHAPTER 3 (PAGE 27) has more on preparing your portfolio and the section in **CHAPTER 6** on 'Portfolio questions' **(PAGE 86)** will cover the questions.

SITUATIONAL QUESTION

QUESTION I

You are the surgical ST and are auditing surgical complications. You notice that your consultant has an unexpectedly large number cases complicated by anastomotic leak. What would you do next?

Positive indicators:

- First, talk to your consultant directly about it.
- If still concerned, talk to the departmental head or clinical director.
- Do not assume blame or gossip.
- Do not remain silent on the issue; report it if still concerned.

PRACTICAL SKILLS

Usually suturing or knot tying. 'Practical skills assessment' in **CHAPTER 5 (PAGE 68)** covers the expected marking scheme.

CLINICAL SCENARIO

A common mistake is to blurt out an operative procedure. For example, if asked about the management of a ruptured aortic aneurysm, don't immediately talk about clamping the aorta! Be systematic and get the basics right: resuscitate, cross-match, call for support, liaise with anaesthetist and theatres. Only then can you get your hands dirty!

There are additional scenarios in the section on Surgery in General **(PAGE I2I)**. My surgical advisors tell me that the scenarios are similar to those for CT1 but you would be expected to perform to a higher standard.

QUESTION I

An acute abdomen (see **CORE MEDICAL TRAINING, CLINICAL SCENARIO 3, PAGE I04**).

QUESTION 2

Management of an unresponsive patient. Surgeons will be expected to know how to manage common medical emergencies (see **ANAESTHESIA, CLINICAL SCENARIO I, PAGE I25**).

REFERENCE

I *The workforce of the future: realistic career planning.* Presentation by Alison Carr, Dean Adviser, MMC (http://www.foundationprogramme.nhs.uk/download.asp?file=alisoncarr.ppt).

Trauma and Orthopaedics

This is one of the most competitive specialties and you have to be the *crème de la crème* to stand a chance. In 2008 there were 54 applicants per training post! At the time of writing (2010) recruitment is local, but a national programme is under consideration. The main entry points into the specialty were at ST1 and ST3.

Career development

HOW TO GET THE EDGE

- Full MRCS
- Attend the courses below
- Present at national or international conferences
- Win national or international prizes
- PhD, MD, or MSc

For ST3, as above plus:

- Record all procedures in a logbook
- Lots of regular assessments, reflective practice, and DOPS

COURSES

Each course you attend will potentially give you a boost at short-listing:

- Basic Surgical Skills
- Care of the Critically Ill Surgical Patient (CCrISP)
- Advanced Trauma Life Support (ATLS)
- AO Principles in Operative Fracture Management Course
- Basic Fracture Management (Royal National Orthopaedic Hospital)
- Basic Techniques in Arthroscopic Surgery (Royal College of Surgeons, England) (CT1 and CT2 applicants)

PRIZES AND PRESENTATIONS

Medical students:

- Same as for Surgery in General (page 119)
- Surgical societies at most medical schools
- Future Orthopaedic Surgeons Prize

Junior doctors: prizes are awarded for presentations (oral or poster) by the following organizations:

- The Association of Surgeons in Training Conference
- British Orthopaedic Research Society

- British Trauma Society
- European Federation of National Associations of Orthopaedics and Traumatology
- British Orthopaedic Association
- Royal Society of Medicine

PUBLICATIONS

- *The Journal of Bone and Joint Surgery*
- *Journal of Orthopaedic Surgery and Research*
- *International Orthopaedics*
- *Arthroscopy, Archives of Orthopaedics and Trauma*
- *Acta Orthopaedica*
- *BMC Musculoskeletal Disorders* (has an article processing fee of over £1000)

Interviews

This is normally in a selection centre with applicants evaluated at several stations. According to the Joint Committee on Surgical Training (JCST), the following assessments have been used in recent years:[1]

- Validation station
- Interview and portfolio
- Situational scenario interview
- 'Motivation for the specialty' interview
- Telephone consultant exercise
- Role-playing scenario (with actor)
- Exercises: written prioritization and case notes
- Practical skills, e.g. suturing

COMMON INTERVIEW QUESTIONS

- What are the attributes of a good team player?
- What are the attributes of a good leader?
- What plans have you followed to develop your understanding of trauma and orthopaedics?
- How do you handle stress?
- Tell me about your research and how it contributes to trauma and orthopaedic practice.

Role-playing scenario

QUESTION I

You are the ST1 on night duty. A patient of yours has been admitted with suspected cauda equina syndrome. There is loss of dorsiflexion in the feet. Both ankle jerks are absent and there is sensory loss on the buttocks. He also has urinary incontinence. Please speak to the consultant radiologist over the phone to request an MRI spine.

Note: Expect the 'radiologist" to be rude, obstructive, and unhelpful. The radiologist may try to persuade you to defer the scan to the next day. If you think a test is urgent you have to be firm and insist. Listen to the radiologist and explain reason behind the urgency. Always be polite and maintain a calm demeanour.

QUESTION 2

An angry pre-operative patient (see **ANAESTHESIA, ROLE-PLAYING SCENARIO 2, PAGE 126**).

Data interpretation

- Blood results of patient with pancreatitis: Ranson, APACHE II scoring
- X-ray interpretation, e.g. abdominal or pelvic film

Situational scenario

QUESTION I

Double trouble with a trauma call (see **SURGERY IN GENERAL, CLINICAL SCENARIO I, PAGE I2I.**)

QUESTION 2

A consultant acting strangely (see **PSYCHIATRY, SITUATIONAL SCENARIO 2, PAGE I44.**)

Clinical scenarios

QUESTION I (STI)

You are the orthopaedic ST1 on-call. The A&E nurse practitioner has referred you an 80-year-old woman who fell in her nursing home. An X-ray confirms a fractured neck of femur. How do you proceed?

Positive indicators:

- Resuscitate as per ATLS
- History, examination, and investigations (bloods, ECG, chest X-ray, lateral X-rays)
- Consider fitness and appropriateness for surgery
- Discuss with patient/ family and consent for procedure
- Nil-by-mouth, IV fluids, thrombo-prophylaxis, mark leg

- Inform senior and discuss in trauma meeting
- Book onto trauma list and inform anaesthetist and ward
- Ortho-geriatric input if required

QUESTION 2 (ST1 OR ST3)

You are the ST1 on-call for surgery. A 25-year-old male pedestrian was hit by a car at 30 mph. The paramedics tell you he has sustained an open tibial fracture. You are the first member of the trauma team to arrive. Two A&E nurses are present. How do you proceed?

Positive indicators:

- Resuscitate as per ATLS
- History and examination (neurovascular status, compartment syndrome and wound size)
- Antibiotics, tetanus prophylaxis, wound dressing, fracture reduction if indicated, splint (plaster above knee back-slab)
- Inform senior, theatres, anaesthetist, plastics or vascular if indicated
- Consent for procedure, nil-by-mouth
- Discuss fixation options (external fixator, intramedullary nail, plate), classification, and recent evidence for above.

QUESTION 3 (ST3)

You are the orthopaedic ST3 on-call. The emergency department have referred you a 6-year-old girl who has sustained an isolated off-ended supracondylar fracture. How do you proceed?

Positive indicators:

- History and examination (neurovascular status, exclude associated injuries)
- Request X-rays (AP/lateral), bloods
- Call paediatricians if suspicion of non-accidental injury
- Above elbow back-slab, analgesia
- Inform senior, theatres and anaesthetist as appropriate
- Consent from parents and explain everything (**important**!)
- Manipulation under anaesthetic, k-wires ± ORIF

TOPICAL QUESTIONS

- Similar to Surgery in General **(PAGE 123)**
- Options and timing of surgery for intracapsular fractured neck of femur in young patients
- Knee arthroscopy, debridement, and washout for osteoarthritis

- Extracapsular hip fracture fixation: DHS versus nailing
- Management of off-ended supracondylar elbow fractures in children

REFERENCE

1 JCST Good Practice Toolkit, Phase 3: Selection Centre Guidance. Joint Committee on Surgical Training, London (www.jcst.org).

Otolaryngology (ENT)

ENT is popular among many trainees because of the variety of patient ages and operation types. It offers work–life balance with on-calls from home and there is considerable private practice work available. Recruitment to ENT (Otolaryngology) is coordinated nationally by a single deanery. Entry is at ST3 and a small number of posts become available each year. In 2008 there were 14 applicants per post.

Career development

HOW TO GET AHEAD

- Try to get a rotation with an ENT post.
- Get published many times. Try to be first author.
- Present at a national meeting which will get you an abstract in a journal.
- Poster presentation. Relatively easy to present at conferences.

COURSES

Same as for Surgery in General (page 119). Here are some additional desirable courses:

- Temporal bone courses
- Sinus surgery courses
- Head and neck surgery/anatomy courses
- ENT radiology courses
- Teach the Teachers/management/leadership courses

PRIZES AND PRESENTATIONS

- Regional otolaryngology meetings: these meetings are generally much easier to present at as a junior doctor and is normally a good stepping-stone to presenting at the national meetings:
  - North of England Otolaryngology Society (www.noeent.com)

- Scottish Otolaryngological Society (www.scottish-otolaryngological-society. scot.nhs.uk)
- The Midland Institute of Otology (www.mio.org.uk)
- The South West ENT Academic Meeting (www.sweam.org.uk)
- The Semon Club: London-based 'case report' meeting. The better presentations are mentioned in the *Journal of Laryngology and Otology*.
- The Royal Society of Medicine: annual essay prize that pre-ST3 junior doctors may enter. Meetings are typically divided into the Otology section and the Laryngology and Rhinology section.
- Otorhinolaryngological Research Society (www.ors.uk.net). Their biannual meeting is an opportunity to present research papers. There are prizes that are specifically for pre-ST3 junior doctors.
- British Rhinological Society Meeting. Interesting audits can be accepted as oral presentations although the standard is high.

JOURNALS

- *Journal of Laryngology and Otology*: accepts case reports, but quality research is more likely to be accepted.
- *The Otolaryngologist*: historically, aimed at the trainees and so acceptance for publication was easier. Due to be revived in the future.
- *Clinical Otolaryngology*: there is competition to get published. Consider the '12 Minute Consultation' section.

Selection centre

In 2010 applicants were assessed at six stations. Below is a sample format:

- Interview: portfolio, commitment to specialty
- Clinical scenario
- Practical skills assessment
- Interview: audit, research, teaching
- Role-playing scenario
- Structured interview: management, leadership, problem solving

CLINICAL SCENARIO

You could be asked about the management of the following surgical scenarios:

- Traumatic nasal epistaxis with severe haemorrhage. Suggestion: resuscitate, consider a lynch incision.
- Post-tonsillectomy haemorrhage. Suggestion: resuscitate, nil-by-mouth, consider options, e.g. observation (if bleeding stops), silver nitrate cauterization, pressure with Magills forceps and adrenaline, theatre.

- Retro-orbital haemorrhage? Suggestion: be aware of potential for blindness, involve ophthalmology, consider mannitol, high-dose steroids, lateral canthotomy.
- Post-oesophagoscopy patient complaining of chest pain. Suggestion: resuscitate, differentiate Boerhaave's syndrome (raised temperature, surgical emphysema, and Hamman's crunch) from a myocardial infarction (cardiac-type pain, ECG changes).

PRACTICAL SKILLS

Here are some tasks previous applicants have had. If these skills are new to you, ask your seniors to show you.

- Assemble a laryngoscope and visualize the cords on a resuscitation dummy. Suggestion: practice with a laryngoscope and a dummy. Take care not to 'click' the dummy (breaking teeth).
- Set up a microscope (that is unbalanced, tightened, and with a non-functioning light). Suggestion: Learn how to balance and loosen a microscope.
- Grommet insertion (in a plastic model). Suggestion: be able to tell which ear is represented and where to insert a grommet (inferior anterior quadrant).
- Tonsil: bleeding vessel tie. Suggestion: know how to use a Negus pusher.

ROLE-PLAYING SCENARIOS

- Explain to a mother whose son has recently been discovered to have profound congenital sensorineural deafness on the right side what can be done. She has read about a cochlear implant in the *Daily Mail*. Suggestion: implants are indicated only in the bilaterally deaf.
- Show how you would deal with an angry patient who has had his operation cancelled and wants to see the consultant (who is in theatre and unable to be contacted).

PROBLEM SOLVING SCENARIO

- You are asked to do extra clinics during theatre sessions because your consultant has frequently been on 'sick leave'. What would you do?

TOPICAL QUESTIONS

- NICE guidelines versus TARGET trial data on management for glue ear in children.
- Indications for scanning a patient with a vestibular schwannoma.
- Do you think a sub-consultant grade post should be created?

Ophthalmology

Ophthalmology offers a combination of medicine and surgery with opportunities for delicate microsurgery. At the time of writing, recruitment for ophthalmology was local. Entry is at ST1 into a run-through programme. Entry at higher levels is occasionally available depending on vacancies in individual deaneries. In 2008 there were 19 applicants per ST1 post.

Career development

How to get ahead

- Present at the Royal College of Ophthalmology (RCOphth) congress
- Pass the part 1 FRCOphth exam
- Win an ophthalmology prize

Courses

- Edinburgh Focus: a recommended foundation course in ophthalmology
- RCOphth basic microsurgical skills course

Prizes and presentations

- The Royal College of Ophthalmology Annual Congress: opportunities to present audits and research projects (posters or oral). Trainees are encouraged to attend and participate.
- Duke-Elder Exam: a prestigious prize for medical students. Sitting the paper would show your interest.
- The Royal Society of Medicine hosts an annual meeting to present cases in ophthalmology (prizes awarded).
- Patrick Trevor-Roper Undergraduate Travel Award: student elective bursary.
- Many medical schools award their own ophthalmology exam.

Journals

- *Eye News*: an opportunity to write an original article, though it is not a peer-reviewed publication.
- *Eye* or the *British Journal of Ophthalmology* are worth subscribing to, but getting published here is much harder.
- *BMC Ophthalmology*: there is a fee exceeding £1000 but it publishes many cases and research papers.

Selection centre

The format differs for each deanery, but previous applicants describe a mixture of interviews and Objective Structured Clinical Examination (OSCE)-style stations. Here is a sample format:

- Portfolio station
- Structured interview: research, commitment to specialty, difficult scenario
- Practical skills assessment
- Clinical scenario

PORTFOLIO STATION

Inspection of portfolio including work-based assessments. Documents from the Royal College of Ophthalmology have attracted particular attention in the past, e.g. Duke-Elder Exam, RCOphth Congress certificate.

PAPER REVIEW

Some applicants have been asked to critically appraise a paper followed by questions on statistics.

PRACTICAL SKILLS

- Suturing skills station
- Microsurgery: eye–hand coordination test with simulator

CLINICAL SCENARIOS

Be prepared for a wide variety of clinical scenarios either in ophthalmology or in general medicine. Often scenarios may lead to an ethics or team-work related dilemma. Examples include:

- How would you approach discussing the result of a Chlamydia-positive swab to a patient with chronic conjunctivitis? Discuss treatment.
- A 16-year-old girl is referred to the eye casualty clinic with headaches and papilloedema. What would you do?
- You are in casualty clinic, a patient presents with sudden loss of vision in one eye. He is very worried. What would you do?

PROBLEM SOLVING SCENARIOS

- You note that a colleague has prescribed the wrong treatment to a patient. How would you handle the situation?
- What would you do if you have concerns that a colleague is putting patients at risk?

- Your consultant is off sick. The clinic is very busy and running late. A patient is angry that he has been waiting for a long time to be seen. You've seen him, but you are not sure what his diagnosis is. What do you do next?

TOPICAL QUESTIONS

- Effect of the NICE glaucoma guidelines on service provision
- Health care equality and the treatment of age-related macular degeneration

Neurosurgery

So you want to be a brain surgeon? (sorry, no more clichés!) In 2008 and 2009, there were between five and six applicants per post. This suggests that neurosurgery is less competitive than other surgical specialties.

Entry is at ST1, ST2, or ST3. The training is 'run-through', i.e. until completion of specialist training. For England, Scotland, and Wales, recruitment is via a single national process. The final hurdle is a selection centre.

Career development

Show your interest by attending or participating in the meetings below. Organize a taster and attend theatre or outpatients. It helps if you have audits, publications, prizes, and research related to neurosurgery.

COURSES

- Advanced Trauma Life Support (ATLS)
- Basic Surgical Skills
- Care of the Critically Ill Surgical Patient (CCrISP)

PRIZES AND PRESENTATION

- Society of British Neurological Surgeons (SBNS) meeting: trainees can co-present with a full member of the SBNS. There is the potential to win prizes.
- Royal Society of Medicine neurosciences meetings: attendance would demonstrate interest.

PUBLICATIONS

- British Journal of Neurosurgery: accepts case reports and series
- Journal of Neurology, Neurosurgery and Psychiatry

Selection centre

Applicants have been selected using a mixture of assessment methods. Each station lasts 10–15 minutes.[1] A sample format is as follows:

- Portfolio interview
- Management interview
- Clinical scenarios
- Image interpretation exercise
- Telephone consultation exercise
- Role-playing scenario
- Practical skills assessment

PORTFOLIO INTERVIEW

- Tell me about an audit you have been involved with.
- Why do you want to do neurosurgery?
- What do you think are the difficulties/challenges for trainees in neurosurgery?

MANAGEMENT INTERVIEW

- How would you cope with a colleague who was drunk at work?
- Do you think that neurosurgery is stressful? How would you cope with the stress?
- Can you think of a situation that you found particularly challenging at work?

CLINICAL SCENARIOS

Follow the advice in **CHAPTER 6, PAGE 90**.

QUESTION 1 (ST1–ST3)

How would you manage a post-operative (neurosurgery) patient with a dropping GCS and in status epilepticus?

Suggestion: Possible intracranial haematoma. Resuscitate, getting assistance, seizure control, and investigating the cause. For ST3+ you would be expected to deliver a more comprehensive explanation of the surgical procedure and long-term management.

QUESTION 2 (ST3)

A 77-year-old man presented with a headache. A CT brain shows a large, acute, sub-dural haematoma with mid-line shift. The A&E doctor has called to refer the patient and ask for advice. The patient on arrival had a GCS of 14 but it is now 8. His blood pressure has been rising and his pupils are dilated unilaterally. The doctor provides a minimal history and asks if you want to give mannitol. What would you do?

Suggestion: Resuscitate, be systematic and logical.

TELEPHONE EXERCISE

There are many possible permutations. You might have to speak to a 'radiologist', 'neurosurgeon', or 'A&E consultant' played by an assessor. Also read **CHAPTER 5, PAGE 80** for more on telephone exercises.

QUESTION 1

Speak to the consultant for Neuro-ITU and ask for a bed for one of your patients. The consultant could challenge you on the appropriateness of your referral or that he would like to 'reserve' his remaining ITU bed.

QUESTION 2

Speak to the neurosurgical consultant on-call (a locum) to come in to help you with an operation that you are not competent with. The procedure is urgent but the consultant might try to persuade you to postpone it.

ROLE-PLAYING SCENARIOS

QUESTION 1

A 35-year-old woman has had an MRI brain for recurrent headaches. It shows a meningioma and your consultant recommends a resection. You are to explain the diagnosis & treatment plan to her.

QUESTION 2

Describe the procedure to and consent a patient for an elective carpal tunnel decompression.

PRACTICAL SKILLS ASSESSMENT

Below are a few of the tasks that previous applicants have had.[1,2] **CHAPTER 5, PAGE 68** has more on practical assessments.

- Surgical knot tying and suturing
- Simulated brain biopsy
- Application of haemostatic (Raney) clips
- Stereoscopic vision test (pilot)
- Microsurgery: removal of beads under microscopy (pilot)

TOPICAL QUESTIONS

- Impact of the European Working Time Directive (EWTD) on neurosurgical training (for trainees and consultants)

- The role of drains in chronic sub-dural haematomas (evidence-based discussion)
- The role of decompressive craniectomy in stroke (indications, evidence)

REFERENCES

1 JCST Good Practice Toolkit, Phase 3: Selection Centre Guidance. Joint Committee on Surgical Training, London (www.jcst.org)

2 Kamaly-Asl, I.D. *et al.* (2009). Testing of practical skills in neurosurgery national selection [abstract]. *British Journal of Neurosurgery*, **23**(5), 471.

Plastic Surgery

Plastic Surgery is more than just aesthetics. Much of it is reconstructive, restoring form and function. Attention to detail and manual dexterity are essential. Because of the small number of training posts, it is fiercely competitive with 23 applicants per post in 2008. Entry is mainly at ST3. Recruitment is national, with the best performing candidates being allocated the deanery of their choice.

Career development

How to get the edge

The advice is the same as for Surgery in General **(PAGE 118)**. As a medical student, apply for one of the electives or bursaries below. Junior doctors should join one of the organizations below and participate in the meetings. Publications and presentations relating to the specialty will demonstrate your interest.

Courses

As for Surgery in General **(PAGE 118)**. The courses listed below would be desirable:

- Emergency management of severe burns, British Burn Association
- Specialty skills in plastic surgery, Royal College of Surgeons of England (RCSeng)
- Basic skills in hand surgery, RCSeng or British Society for Surgery of the Hand (BSSH)
- Elective skills in facial trauma, RCSeng

Prizes and presentations

- British Association of Plastic Reconstructive and Aesthetic Surgeons (BAPRAS): junior doctors can present posters at their biannual meetings.

For medical students, there is an excellent careers day and bursaries for electives.

- The BSSH: student elective bursary and Mr R G Pulvertaft (essay) Medal. There are opportunities to present (posters) and win prizes at the scientific meetings.
- British Burn Association Annual Meeting: poster and oral presentations with the potential for winning prizes.
- ASiT-PLASTA Prize for the best abstracts presented at the Association of Surgeons in Training (ASiT) conference.

Interviews

The selection centre consists of a mixture of interviews and OSCE-style stations. According to the Joint Committee on Surgical Training (JCST), selection centres have consisted of the following:[1]

- Structured interview, e.g. audit, teaching, and research
- Portfolio interview
- Telephone consultant
- Role-playing scenario
- Paper review exercise
- Clinical scenario and discussion

PORTFOLIO STATION

- Do you have a specialist interest in any area of plastic surgery and why?
- Inspection of logbook and work-based assessments.
- What have you learned from your case-based discussions?
- Why do want to do plastic surgery?
- Do you have a specialist interest in any area of plastic surgery and why?

ROLE-PLAYING SCENARIOS

Some suitable practice scenarios are given in **CHAPTER 6**.

CLINICAL SCENARIOS

QUESTION I

You are called to the high-dependency unit to see a persistently hypotensive 73-year-old man who is 2 hours post-op (intra-oral free flap reconstruction for tumour excision). How would you proceed? How do you assess a free flap?

QUESTION 2

You are the plastics registrar asked to review a 57-year-old man involved in a road traffic accident. He has a significant degloving injury with cold and pale digits. There is no radial pulse palpable. What are you next steps? How long is the critical ischemia period?

QUESTION 3

You are called to the ward to see a 47-year-old woman who is 5 hours post-op. She had undergone a bilateral breast reduction. She now has increasing pain and swelling in her right breast. How would you proceed?

QUESTION 4

How would you manage a 60-year-old man with full-thickness burn? How do you estimate the percentage of skin involved? Calculate the fluid resuscitation requirements.

TELEPHONE SCENARIO

More advice is given on telephone scenarios in **CHAPTER 5**.

QUESTION 1

You are the plastics ST3 on-call and it is midnight. A 45-year-old patient has necrotizing fasciitis in her right lower limb. You have 5 minutes to read the notes and formulate a plan. You are then to call your consultant Mr Gruff with your plan. [Note: Do not expect Mr Gruff to be friendly. He may be off-putting on purpose.]

Positive indicators:

- Clear communication
- Resuscitation and sensible plan
- Teamwork, i.e. anaesthetist, theatres, juniors
- Be firm with a 'difficult' consultant

PAPER-REVIEW EXERCISE

You could be given a paper to critically appraise. Revise your evidence-based medicine and ensure that the evidence is applicable to your patients' circumstances.

TOPICAL QUESTIONS

Similar to Surgery in General (page 123) plus the following:

- Face transplantation: the ethics involved.
- Cosmetic versus reconstructive surgery
- Should plastics surgeons be performing primary resection for breast cancer?

REFERENCE

1 JCST Good Practice Toolkit, Phase 3: Selection Centre Guidance. Joint Committee on Surgical Training, London (www.jcst.org)

Acute Medicine

This is a young and growing specialty. It is anticipated that consultant numbers (and training posts) will be expanded. Historically, it is less competitive than other medical specialties though this fluctuates from year to year. From 2011, recruitment will be organized centrally by the RCP.

Career development

HOW TO GET THE EDGE

- Present at the Society of Acute Medicine
- Get published
- Show an interest in Acute Medicine early on

COURSES

- Advanced Life Support (ALS)
- IMPACT (Ill Medical Patients' Acute Care and Treatment) course
- University College London medical emergencies course for trainee doctors
- Royal College of Physicians Advances in Acute Medicine (training day)

PRIZES AND PRESENTATIONS

- Society of Acute Medicine: hosts biannual meetings where trainees are encouraged to present (oral and poster). Prizes are awarded for the best presentations.
- See the section on CMT **(PAGE 111)** for other suitable opportunities.

JOURNALS

As for CMT **(PAGE 111)** and Emergency Medicine **(PAGE 128)**.

Interviews

The format varies from deanery to deanery but is predominantly interview-based. A typical interview consists of three interview stations each lasting 10–12 minutes:

- Interview 1: portfolio, achievements, commitment to specialty
- Interview 2 : research, audit, problem solving scenario
- Interview 3: role-playing scenario

ROLE-PLAYING SCENARIOS

Examples include breaking bad news and discussing 'do not resuscitate' orders. **THE SECTION IN CHAPTER 5 'ROLE-PLAYING SCENARIO' (PAGE 71)** has more practice scenarios.

QUESTION I

Consent a patient for thrombolysis (see **EMERGENCY MEDICINE, ROLE-PLAYING SCENARIO I, PAGE I32.**)

QUESTION 2

An anxious patient on the wards (see **CARDIOLOGY, ROLE-PLAYING SCENARIO I, PAGE I70.**)

QUESTION 3

Patient education with an asthmatic patient (see **RESPIRATORY ROLE-PLAYING SCENARIO I, PAGE I81**).

QUESTION 4

A patient who wants to self-discharge (see **RESPIRATORY, ROLE-PLAYING SCENARIO 2, PAGE I82.**)

CLINICAL SCENARIOS

Go through the clinical scenarios in the section on CMT **(PAGE II3)**. Because you are applying for ST3, you will be expected to perform at a higher standard. Below are a couple of additional scenarios.

QUESTION I

An unresponsive patient on the medical ward (see **ANAESTHESIA, CLINICAL SCENARIO I, PAGE I25.**)

QUESTION 2

An emergency with a diagnostic challenge (see **ENDOCRINOLOGY, CLINICAL SCENARIO I, PAGE I74**).

QUESTION 3

How would you manage a young woman with liver failure after a paracetamol overdose.

Suggestion: Supportive care, regular monitoring if clotting, albumin, pH, and lactate. Involve the hepatologists early on. Have a good understanding of capacity and sectioning under the Mental Health Act.

QUESTION 4

Recognition and management of a patient with septic arthritis.

Suggestion: Have a high degree of suspicion. Urgent joint aspiration and antibiotic therapy is key. Involve the surgeons as soon as possible.

QUESTION 5

How well do you know pneumothorax? (see **RESPIRATORY, CLINICAL SCENARIO 3, PAGE 182**).

TOPICAL QUESTIONS

- Discuss the burden of alcohol on the NHS and society. How would you deal with this?
- There is an increasing call for the presence of Acute Medicine consultants during out-of-hours. Is this a good thing?
- The organization of outpatient services for acute medical care, e.g. outpatient intravenous antibiotic therapy, deep venous thrombosis clinics.

Cardiology

Cardiology is a research-led specialty with plenty of high-tech gadgets and practical procedures. In 2010 there were 14 applicants for each post. Entry is at ST3 and recruitment is led nationally by the Royal College of Physicians (RCP).

Career development

Successful candidates must demonstrate their commitment to the specialty. Research is a popular route, with many trainees holding an MD or PhD. Others build on their clinical experience by taking up LATs (locum appointment—training) or 'clinical fellow' posts. Having practical skills relevant to Cardiology is a plus on the person specifications. Don't worry if you can't deploy an intra-coronary stent! Get experience in echocardiography, cardioversion, or chest pain clinics instead.

PRIZES AND PRESENTATIONS

- British Cardiovascular Society (BCS): an opportunity to present (poster) and win a prize if lucky.
- Royal Society of Medicine (RSM): hosts an annual meeting for budding cardiologists to present research and audit.

PUBLICATIONS

- *British Journal of Cardiology*: accepts review articles, research and letters
- *Cardiology News*: accepts review articles and letters
- *Clinical Cardiology*: accepts case reports, research, and articles

COURSES

- BCS: organizes courses such as the Cardiology Review Course
- RCP: hosts regular seminars relating to cardiology
- RSM: regular Cardiology Section meetings
- British Society of Echocardiography: directory of echocardiography courses

Interviews

Below is a recently used interview format consisting of three stations each of 15 minutes' duration:

- Station 1: portfolio, commitment to specialty, skills, clinical experience
- Station 2: clinical scenario (discussion)
- Station 3: situational scenario, clinical governance, research

ROLE-PLAYING SCENARIOS

QUESTION 1

A young man on the Cardiology Ward presented with a 'sharp' chest pain and saddle-shaped ST elevation on his ECG. Your consultant diagnosed pericarditis and thinks he is well enough to be discharged. Explain the diagnosis to the patient and its implications. [Actor brief: You had terrible chest pain a few days ago. Your father died of a heart attack and you are terrified you had one. The doctor in A&E said you had an abnormal 'heart tracing'.]

Suggestion: Explore his fears and be reassuring.

QUESTION 2

You are in clinic with a patient who had an ST elevation myocardial infarction and a drug-eluting stent last month. He continues to smoke and frequently misses his medications. Explain to him the importance of compliance.

CLINICAL SCENARIOS

QUESTION 1

A previously well 55-year-old man with hypertension and high cholesterol (but no other risk factors) presented the day before with chest pain. Serial ECGs have been unremarkable and his 12-hour troponin is negative. How would you proceed?

Suggestion: A thorough history is provides much of the diagnostic information. Know the 2010 NICE guidelines on chest pain and the recommended investigations. A stress ECG is **no longer** recommended to diagnose ischaemia.

QUESTION 2

A 40-year-old man presents with 2 weeks of breathlessness. An echocardiogram shows a markedly dilated left ventricle with severe left ventricular dysfunction. How would you manage this patient?

Suggestion: History: viral illness, alcohol history, family. Examination and further investigations, e.g. blood tests, angiography, cardiac MRI.

TOPICAL QUESTIONS

- NICE guidelines often generate much discussion. Be up to date on the latest ones, i.e. chest pain and acute coronary syndrome.
- Are targets for the Cardiology Clinic a good thing (i.e. the 6-week rule)?
- Should cardiologists be part of the general medical on-call?

Care of the Elderly (Geriatrics)

This is one of the few medical specialties with a generalist approach. Recruitment is organized nationally by the Royal College of Physicians. The highest-scoring candidates are interviewed by the deanery of their choice. Of the medical specialties, Care of the Elderly has the largest number of training jobs, with five applicants for each post.

Career development

COURSES

- The Royal College of Physicians (RCP) (London and Edinburgh) organize regular seminars relevant to Geriatrics
- Royal Society of Medicine (RSM): Alex Comfort lecture

PRIZES AND PRESENTATIONS

- British Geriatrics Society: awards essay prizes to medical students. Its annual meeting is an opportunity for trainees to present (www.bgs.org.uk)
- European Union Geriatric Medicine Society: its annual meeting is an opportunity to present cases and research (www.eugms.org)
- RSM: hosts an annual meeting to present cases relating to Care of the Elderly with the chance to win prizes. There is an annual essay prize
- Faculty of the Psychiatry of Old Age (of the Royal College of Psychiatrists): poster presentation and prize

Publications

- *Geriatric Medicine*: if you have an idea for a review article, this is the place
- *BMC Geriatrics*: accepts cases and research but there is a fee in excess of £1000
- *Age and ageing*: a well-known journal that accept case reports, letters, and articles
- *European Geriatric Medicine*: a newly established journal on the look-out for cases, research, and letters

Interviews

In recent years interviews have followed a three-station format:

- Station 1: portfolio station, commitment to specialty, clinical experience, and skills
- Station 2: clinical scenario (discussion) or role-playing scenario
- Station 3: situational scenario (discussion)

Role-playing scenarios

- Explain to an anxious daughter about the insertion of a PEG tube for her mother, an inpatient on the stroke ward.
- Speak to family about a 'do not resuscitate' order for an elderly patient from a nursing home who has severe pneumonia.

CLINICAL SCENARIOS

QUESTION 1

You are in clinic. An elderly patient has a new diagnosis of Parkinson's disease and is struggling to manage at home alone. How would you manage him?

Suggestion: NICE guidelines on Parkinson's disease, assess social situation, additional support if required, fully involve patient and family.

QUESTION 2

A patient attends the falls clinic with a history of recurrent collapses at home. How would you proceed?

Suggestion: NICE guidelines on falls assessment, multidisciplinary approach.

SITUATIONAL SCENARIO

QUESTION 1

An 82-year-old patient with severe Alzheimer's is admitted from a nursing home with dehydration and anorexia. She is usually bed-bound and dependent on carers for everything. She repeatedly pulls out IV lines or nasogastric tubes. Her family feel strongly that she should be fed with a PEG tube. They say she was deeply religious and would never have contemplated taking her own life. What would you do?

Suggestion: There often is no 'correct' answer. Consider referral to psychogeriatrician and discuss at the multidisciplinary team (MDT) meeting. Family should always be consulted and their views considered. However, it is the doctor who ultimately has to decide.

QUESTION 2

An elderly patient was admitted with a urinary tract infection. Your consultant assessed her on the ward round and thinks she is ready for discharge. However, the patient's daughter is unhappy with this. She feels the patient is confused and is concerned for her safety.

Suggestion: Speak to the daughter and explore her concerns, involve other professionals, e.g. nurses, physiotherapist, occupational therapist, social worker. Consider reassessing the patient.

TOPICAL QUESTIONS

- The challenges an ageing population presents to the NHS.
- Know the latest NICE guidelines: falls, Parkinson's disease, stroke.
- Funding for dementia patients: should this be from the NHS or social services?

Endocrinology

Recruitment for England, Scotland, and Wales is hosted by the Royal College of Physicians (RCP). Applicants apply online and short-listed candidates attend interview at the deanery of their choice. Entry is at ST3 and there were six applicants for every training post in 2010.

Career development

HOW TO GET AHEAD

- Attend endocrinology clinics and talk to trainees
- Get involved in related audits
- Attend and participate in the meetings below

PRIZES AND PRESENTATIONS

- Society for Endocrinology: annual clinical updates are an opportunity to present cases. The society awards additional prizes to undergraduates and junior doctors.

- Diabetes UK Conference: an excellent platform to give verbal and poster presentations with an opportunity for prizes.
- Hammersmith Multidisciplinary Endocrine Symposium: opportunity to present cases and win prizes.

COURSES

- Advanced Life Support (ALS), Acute Life-threatening Events—Recognition and Treatment (ALERT), Ill Medical Patients' Acute Care and Treatment (IMPACT) certification
- Observer at a DAFNE course (Dose Adjustment for Normal Eating; an educational programme for patients with type 1 diabetes). This would show your interest

JOURNALS

- *Clinical Endocrinology*
- *Diabetes Medicine*
- *Practical Diabetes International*

Interviews

Previous interviews have consisted of three stations, each lasting 10 minutes:

- Station 1: portfolio, commitment to specialty, audit, research
- Station 2: clinical scenario (discussion)
- Station 3: clinical scenario, audit, previous critical incidents

COMMON INTERVIEW QUESTIONS

- Demonstrate your interest in Endocrinology.
- What teaching experience do you have and how would you improve it further?
- Tell me about your research project and what you have gained from it.
- How would you deal with a critical incident involving yourself?
- Tell us any article you have read recently which has changed your clinical practice.

CLINICAL SCENARIO

QUESTION I

You are the on-call registrar and have been asked to see an 18-year-old woman presenting with vomiting and generalized abdominal pain. She was previously diagnosed with hypothyroidism and takes levothyroxine regularly. She has no other illnesses or drugs. On examination, she appears tanned. She is apyrexial, tachycardic and hypotensive but has normal oxygen saturations. She has been given 2 L of IV colloid. Blood results do not suggest sepsis and her glucose is 3.5 mmol/L. How will you proceed?

Positive indicators:

- Resuscitate!
- Investigations: urea and electrolytes, random cortisol, ACTH
- Think Addison's disease: empirically hydrocortisone

QUESTION 2

See the scenario concerning diabetic ketoacidosis in Question 4 in the section on CMT (PAGE 114).

TOPICAL QUESTIONS

- The vertical integration of primary and secondary care in diabetes
- The increasing role of nurse practitioners in endocrinology. Good or bad?
- Metabolic syndrome

SOURCE OF INFORMATION

The Society of Endocrinology (www.endocrinology.org).

Gastroenterology

Recruitment in England and Wales is centralized and hosted by the Royal College of Physicians (RCP) (London). Applications are via an online portal with a shared short-listing methodology. The interview process has been standardized across deaneries. In 2010, it was estimated that there were eight applicants per post.

Career development

HOW TO GET THE EDGE

- Show an interest: get involved with conferences and presentations
- Attend endoscopy and talk to gastroenterology trainees
- Attend clinics and multidisciplinary team (MDT) meetings

COURSES

The British Society of Gastroenterology (BSG) and RCP host relevant conferences and seminars. Attendance at a few of these will show your interest. If you have extra cash, attendance at a JAG (Joint Advisory Group on GI Endoscopy) Basic Skills Course in Endoscopy is desirable, though not essential.

PRIZES AND PRESENTATIONS

The BSG Annual Meeting is an opportunity to present your poster and win a prize.

PUBLICATIONS

- *BMC Gastroenterology* publishes many case reports but there is a fee exceeding £1000
- *Frontline Gastroenterology*
- *British Journal of Nutrition*
- *Gut*
- *Alimentary Pharmacology and Therapeutics*

Interviews

Interviews have been standardized to a three-station format:

- Station 1: portfolio, commitment, and suitability to specialty
- Station 2: discussion of two clinical scenarios
- Station 3: presentation followed by questions

COMMON INTERVIEW QUESTIONS

- What makes you suited to the specialty?
- What have you done outside of work to learn about Gastroenterology?
- Tell me about a related paper that has changed your practice.

ROLE-PLAYING SCENARIOS

The following are possible scenarios at future interviews.

QUESTION I

Breaking bad news at endoscopy: upper gastrointestinal malignancy.

QUESTION 2

Counsel a patient who drinks excessively on safe alcohol consumption.

CLINICAL SCENARIOS

QUESTION I

How do you manage a patient with hepatic encephalopathy?

Suggestion: Assess severity, identify and treat the cause, management, e.g. lactulose, rifaximin, involve hepatologists.

QUESTION 2

Managing variceal bleeding (see Core Medical Training, PAGE 113).

QUESTION 3

Managing liver failure in paracetamol overdose (see Acute Medicine, **PAGE 168**).

PRESENTATIONS

Previous applicants have been assessed on three main areas:

- The ability to answer questions (listen and answer precisely)
- Generic presentational skills
- Topic choice and relevance

Choose a topic related to Gastroenterology that you are interested in. Make sure you understand the topic well as it will help you when answering questions.

TOPICAL QUESTIONS

- Bowel cancer screening: which patients are eligible, how the screening works.
- Global Rating Scale for evaluating endoscopy suites.
- Be aware of recent guidelines, i.e. irritable bowel syndrome (NICE), variceal haemorrhage in cirrhotic patients (BSG).

SOURCE OF INFORMATION

The British Society of Gastroenterology (www.bsg.org.uk).

Infectious Disease

At the time of writing (2010) recruitment was held locally. Entry is at ST3. In 2007, there were nine applicants per post.

Career development

COURSES

- Ill Medical Patients' Acute Care and Treatment (IMPACT)
- Diploma in Tropical Medicine and Hygiene
- Diploma in Hospital Infection Control

PRIZES AND PRESENTATIONS

The following societies host regular meetings with opportunities to present and win prizes:

- Royal Society of Infectious Diseases: medical student and trainee prizes.
- British Infection Society: there is an annual 'trainee day' with an opportunity to present and win a prize

- British HIV Association
- Federation of Infection Societies
- British Association for Sexual Health and HIV

PUBLICATIONS

- *BMC infectious Diseases*
- *HIV Medicine*
- *Transactions of the Royal Society of Tropical Medicine and Hygiene*
- *International Health*

Interviews

The interviews vary with each deanery. Previous applicants have reported the questions in the following areas to be common: topical issues; portfolio; motivation for choosing the specialty.

COMMON QUESTIONS

- What recent changes in human behaviour have influenced disease?
- What do you see as the future of the Infectious Disease specialty?
- What is the trend of MRSA rates in the UK at the moment?
- What infectious disease story have you read about in the news?

ROLE-PLAYING SCENARIOS

- Consenting a patient for a HIV test.
- Taking a sexual history from a patient.

CLINICAL SCENARIOS

- A 25-year-old female presents with fever and haemoptysis. Describe the differential diagnosis and your initial management plan.
- A 30-year-old man returned from West Africa 1 week ago. He was a volunteer in a village school. He is pyrexial, tachycardic, and hypotensive. How would you manage him?

TOPICAL QUESTIONS

- Public access to oseltamivir for 'swine flu' without prescription.
- Flu pandemics.
- Hospital acquired infections, e.g. *Clostridium difficile*.
- The use of routine HIV testing in parts of the UK (cost implications).

Renal

The longevity of relationships with renal patients coupled with the acute and esoteric presentations of renal disease make renal medicine particularly appealing. Recruitment throughout England and Wales is hosted by the Royal College of Physicians via a single application process. Short-listed candidates will be interviewed by deaneries following a standardized format. In 2010, there were six applicants per training post.

Career development

HOW TO GET THE EDGE

Show commitment by spending time on a renal ward, renal clinic, and dialysis unit. If possible, try to observe a live donor kidney transplant operation. The Renal SpR Club hosts biannual meetings for registrars but will welcome keen core medical trainees; contact the committee's local representative.

PRIZES AND PRESENTATIONS

The Renal Association offers bursaries for electives and for trainees to attend the association's annual meeting. There is an opportunity to present at the annual meeting.

COURSES

Advanced Life Support (ALS) is a must whilst Acute Life-threatening Events—Recognition and Treatment (ALERT) and Ill Medical Patients' Acute Care and Treatment (IMPACT) certification are desirable. Equality and Diversity training is also desirable. You can complete training online via an 'e-course'.

PUBLICATIONS

- *Nephron*
- *Nephrology Dialysis Transplantation*
- *British Journal of Renal Medicine*
- *Journal of Renal Care*
- *Journal of Renal Nutrition*

Interviews

Recent interviews have had two interview stations of 15 minutes each:

- Station 1: portfolio, commitment to specialty, clinical governance, research
- Station 2: clinical scenario

Role-playing scenarios

You could be asked about the following scenarios:

- Explaining to a patient (or family) with end-stage renal failure about end-of-life care or withdrawal from dialysis.
- Explaining renal replacement therapy options to a patient with established renal failure.
- Describe the members and their roles in a renal multidisciplinary team.

Clinical scenarios

Applicants are expected to know 'the basics of managing renal disease and renal emergencies'. A common renal emergency is an 'acute kidney injury' scenario. Also be aware of the pros and cons of different renal replacement therapy options.

QUESTION 1

A&E have referred to you an 80-year-old lady found on the floor by neighbours. She had extensive bruising all over her hips and back. X-rays show no fractures but her renal function is markedly deranged (serum urea 22 mmol/L, creatinine 321 µmol/L). Previously she had normal renal function. How would you manage her?

Topical questions

- Do you wish to be an academic or clinical nephrologist? Why and what challenges do you foresee?
- Acute kidney injury (formerly acute renal failure; NCEPOD Report 2009)
- Live kidney donation and directed donation.

Sources of information

- The Renal Association (www.renal.org)
- The Renal SpR Club (www.sprclub.org)

Respiratory

From 2011, recruitment will be organised centrally by the RCP. In 2007 there were 10 applicants per post.

Career development

How to get the edge

Show your commitment to the specialty by attending conferences and getting involved with organizations such as the British Thoracic Society (BTS). Join an educational course if you can.

Courses

- BTS: non-invasive ventilation, radiology course
- Royal College of Physicians (London): chest drain course, respiratory emergencies

Prizes and presentations

- British Thoracic Society: the winter meeting has hundreds of presentations (oral and poster) with the chance for trainees and medical students to win prizes (www.brit-thoracic.org.uk)
- European Respiratory Society Congress: a fantastic opportunity to present internationally. In 2009, over 5000 submissions were received and over 80% were presented.
- Royal Society of Medicine: medical students can apply for elective bursaries.

Publications

- *Thorax*: a prestigious journal that accepts case reports and original research.
- *Chest Medicine On-line*: peer-reviewed electronic journal that accepts case reports, articles, letters. It claims to have 'the fastest submission to publication rate'.
- *BMC Pulmonary Medicine*: peer-reviewed, Medline. Also accepts submissions from trainees, but there is a fee in excess of £1000.
- *The Journal of Respiratory Disease*: case reports and articles.

Interviews

The interview format will vary slightly for each deanery, but a common format is:

- Station 1: portfolio station, commitment to specialty, achievements
- Station 2: teaching, clinical governance, research
- Station 3: situational scenario, teamwork, coping with pressure

Role-playing scenarios

Question I

An 18-year-old man admitted for a severe exacerbation of asthma is to be discharged today. This is his fifth admission in a year. He smokes regularly and is not compliant with his inhalers. Speak to him about ways of improving his asthma control. Is there anything else you want to check?

Suggestion: Education on asthma control, smoking cessation support, check inhaler technique, peak flowmeter use, home and work environment.

An 18-year-old woman presents with acute breathlessness. She is tachypnoeic and her arterial blood gas shows hypoxia with respiratory alkalosis. Your consultant suspects a pulmonary embolus and wants her to be admitted for treatment and a ventilation perfusion scan. The nurses report she is refusing treatment and admission. Speak to her.

Suggestion: Explore her concerns in a non-confrontational manner, explain the dangers of pulmonary embolus without treatment. There may be multiple concerns, e.g. undisclosed pregnancy, illicit drug use, fear of needles.

CLINICAL SCENARIOS

QUESTION 1

You are seeing a 70-year-old man with COPD in the Chest Clinic. He is asking if he can have oxygen at home. How would you asses if long-term oxygen therapy is suitable?

Suggestion: Be aware of the clinical indications.

QUESTION 2

A 68-year-old patient with an exacerbation of COPD on the ward has been increasingly breathless. On examination he has poor air entry and is wheezy with a prolonged expiratory phase. An arterial blood gas shows he is hypoxic with a marked respiratory acidosis. He is already on high-dose steroids and regular nebulizers. How would you proceed?

Suggestion: Consider intravenous theophyllines and critical care, know the indications for non-invasive ventilation.

QUESTION 3

A 20-year-old man, previously well, presents with pleuritic chest pain and breathlessness. His oxygen saturations are 96% and he has a respiratory rate of 16 breaths/min. His blood pressure and heart rate are normal. He has reduced air entry and hyper-resonance in the right chest. His trachea is central. A chest X-ray confirms a pneumothorax with almost complete collapse of his right lung. What do you do?

Suggestion: Read up the BTS guidelines for managing primary pneumothorax. High-flow oxygen, analgesia and aspiration. Repeat chest X-ray. A chest drain is indicated only if repeated aspiration fails.

TOPICAL QUESTIONS

- What do you think of the growing role of respiratory nurse practitioners?
- Recent BTS or NICE guidelines, e.g. asthma, pneumonia, non-invasive ventilation

CHAPTER 8

If at first you don't succeed, try, try again

If you don't get a job offer, don't be too disheartened. You are not alone. Many doctors don't succeed in getting a training job on their first, second, or even third attempt. This is particularly true if it is a competitive specialty. Instead, see this is an opportunity to build your experience and improve yourself for the next round. The most important thing is to learn from your mistakes and move forward.

Back to the drawing board

Use this opportunity to take stock and ask yourself some important questions. There are no correct answers and ultimately it is for you to decide what to do. Think hard and choose carefully.

- For how many years are you willing to keep reapplying (bearing in mind that you have about 30 working years ahead)?
- Would you be willing to commit additional years in research, e.g. PhD, MD?
- Is there another specialty which interests you but is less competitive?
- If recruitment is organized locally, are you able to apply to more deaneries? This can improve your chances of success.
- Is this the right time to try new experiences, e.g. career change, working abroad, travelling?

Try, try again

Persistence and dedication are essential for getting into specialty training. Many specialty trainees I know had applied to the specialty repeatedly. In between applications, they dedicate their spare time working on their CV. If at first you don't succeed, try, try again and improve yourself with each attempt.

Get feedback

You can only improve if you know your weaknesses. Request feedback on your interview from the deanery. Some deaneries give out minimal information. That's no good. You need a detailed breakdown of your short-listing and interview scores.

The Data Protection Act of 1998 allows you to see information held about you. If the feedback you receive is unhelpful, e-mail a formal request 'subject access request' to the deanery. Your e-mail should start with the sentence 'Please send me the information which I am entitled to under the Section 7(1) of the Data Protection Act 1998'. Then describe the information you require in detail.

By law, the deanery has 40 calendar days to comply. If you get no response, contact the Information Commissioner's Office at casework@ico.gsi.gov.uk. Visit their website if you need more information (www.ico.gov.uk).

Improving yourself

1. Use the feedback from the deanery and the career development tool in **CHAPTER 2 (PAGE 9)** to help identify your weak areas. If you were not short-listed, it means that you need to work on your application form. If you made it to the interview, it means your interview skills need polishing, though it wouldn't hurt to spend time improving your CV as well.

2. Seek the advice of trainees and consultants in the specialty. Ask them to review your CV and to give you suggestions on how you can improve for the next round. Write down their advice so you don't forget it—this advice is worth its weight in gold.

3. Set goals and plan. Set long-term and mid-term goals which are specific and realistic. Plan how you are going to achieve your goals. For example, if your goal is to have a publication, break it down into a few different steps. You would have to browse different journals, read the instructions to authors, think of cases you could submit, request patient notes,

and approach the patient for consent etc. Specify how you intend to achieve those goals. Commit your plan to paper.

4. Do it and stick to your plans. Keep the momentum going and don't lose your enthusiasm.

Last but not least, review the advice in this book. Don't forget to read the section on your specialty of interest. I wish you luck on your journey to specialty training. Work hard, work smart, and remember to enjoy the journey.

Appendices

Appendix 1: Deaneries

Publicly available short-list and interview protocols from the following deanery and royal college websites were used as reference material for Chapters 4, 5, 6, and 7. The competition ratios for the specialties quoted in Chapter 7 are from Modernising Medical Careers (www.mmc.nhs.uk).

Deanery websites

East Midlands Healthcare Workforce Deanery
www.eastmidlandsdeanery.nhs.uk

Kent, Surrey and Sussex (KSS) Deanery
www.kssdeanery.org

London Deanery
www.londondeanery.ac.uk

Mersey Deanery
www.merseydeanery.nhs.uk

NHS East of England Multi Professional Deanery
www.eoedeanery.nhs.uk

NHS West Midlands Workforce Deanery
www.westmidlandsdeanery.nhs.uk

North Western Deanery
www.nwpgmd.nhs.uk

Northern Deanery
www.northerndeanery.org

Northern Ireland Medical and Dental Training Agency
www.nimdta.gov.uk

Oxford Deanery
www.oxforddeanery.nhs.uk

Scottish Medical Training
www.scotmt.scot.nhs.uk

Severn Deanery
www.severndeanery.nhs.uk

South West Peninsula Deanery
www.peninsuladeanery.nhs.uk

Wessex Deanery
www.wessexdeanery.nhs.uk

Yorkshire and the Humber Postgraduate Deanery
www.yorksandhumberdeanery.nhs.uk

Appendix 2: Royal college websites

College of Emergency Medicine
www.collemergencymed.ac.uk

Royal College of Anaesthetists
www.rcoa.ac.uk

Royal College of General Practitioners
www.rcgp.org.uk

Royal College of Obstetricians and Gynaecologists
www.rcog.org.uk

Royal College of Ophthalmologists
www.rcophth.ac.uk

Royal College of Paediatrics and Child Health
www.rcpch.ac.uk

Royal College of Physicians
www.rcplondon.ac.uk
www.cmtrecruitment.org.uk
www.st3recruitment.org.uk

Royal College of Psychiatrists
www.rcpsych.ac.uk

Royal College of Radiologists
www.rcr.ac.uk

The Royal College of Surgeons of England
www.rcseng.ac.uk

The UK's Faculty of Public Health
www.fph.org.uk

Appendix 3

Interview practice feedback form

Interviewee name:

Interview question asked:

What was good:

What could have been better:

Suggestions for improvement:

Please score answer:

| Poor | Below average | Average | Good | Outstanding |

Appendix 4

Interview question feedback form

Interviewee name:

Interview question asked:

What was good (i.e. positive indicators demonstrated):

What needs improvement (i.e. positive indicators not demonstrated):

Other suggestions for improvement:

Please score answer:

Poor	Below	Average	Good	Outstanding
1 point	average	3 points	4 points	5 points
	2 points			

Index